Recent Results in Cancer Research

Volume 197

Managing Editors

P. M. Schlag, Berlin, Germany
H.-J. Senn, St. Gallen, Switzerland

Associate Editors

P. Kleihues, Zürich, Switzerland
F. Stiefel, Lausanne, Switzerland
B. Groner, Frankfurt, Germany
A. Wallgren, Göteborg, Sweden

Founding Editor

P. Rentchnik, Geneva, Switzerland

For further volumes:
http://www.springer.com/series/392

Ute Goerling

Editor

Psycho-Oncology

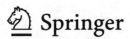 Springer

Editor
Ute Goerling
Department of Psychooncology
Charité Comprehensive Cancer Center
Berlin
Germany

ISSN 0080-0015   ISSN 2197-6767 (electronic)
ISBN 978-3-642-40186-2   ISBN 978-3-642-40187-9 (eBook)
DOI 10.1007/978-3-642-40187-9
Springer Heidelberg New York Dordrecht London

Library of Congress Control Number: 2013953265

Printed on acid-free paper

Springer is part of Springer Science+Business Media (www.springer.com)

Contents

Psychosocial Impact of Cancer.   1
Susanne Singer

Fear of Progression.   11
Peter Herschbach and Andreas Dinkel

Gender Opportunities in Psychosocial Oncology.   31
Matthew Loscalzo and Karen Clark

Psycho-Oncology: A Patient's View   49
Patricia Garcia-Prieto

The Oncological Patient in the Palliative Situation   59
Steffen Eychmueller, Diana Zwahlen and Monica Fliedner

Psychosocial Burden of Family Caregivers to Adults with Cancer. . . .   73
Anna-leila Williams

Rehabilitation for Cancer Patients.   87
Joachim Weis and Jürgen M. Giesler

Cancer Survivorship in Adults. 103
Cecilie E. Kiserud, Alv A. Dahl, Jon Håvard Loge
and Sophie D. Fosså

Psycho-Oncological Interventions and Psychotherapy
in the Oncology Setting 121
Mirjam de Vries and Friedrich Stiefel

Quality of Life in Oncology 137
Ute Goerling and Anna Stickel

Psychosocial Impact of Cancer

Susanne Singer

Abstract

Diagnosis and treatment of malignant diseases affect in many ways the lives of patients, relatives and friends. In this chapter, we summarise the current knowledge concerning the psychosocial consequences of cancer.

Contents

1	Psychological Impact	2
	1.1 Psychological Reaction to the Cancer Diagnosis	2
	1.2 Denial	2
	1.3 Co-morbid Mental Health Conditions	3
	1.4 Potential Positive Impact	4
2	Social Impact	5
	2.1 Socioeconomic Position	5
	2.2 Social Relations	6
References		7

S. Singer (✉)
Epidemiology and Health Services Research, University Medical Centre Mainz, Obere Zahlbacher Straße 69, 55131, Mainz, Germany
e-mail: singers@uni-mainz.de

U. Goerling (ed.), *Psycho-Oncology*, Recent Results in Cancer Research 197,
DOI: 10.1007/978-3-642-40187-9_1, © Springer-Verlag Berlin Heidelberg 2014

1   Psychological Impact

1.1   Psychological Reaction to the Cancer Diagnosis

After a person hears he or she is diagnosed with cancer, the first reaction frequently is a sort of shock: "It can not be me; they must have mixed up the test results with another person". For many patients, receiving such a diagnosis is associated with the fear of intense pain, loss of control, stigmatisation and death (Holland et al. 1989). Getting such a diagnosis therefore feels like a nightmare. Complex processes of denial and subsequent realisation of the truth, often followed by denial again, are seen in those patients.

After a while, depending on the psychosocial resources a patient has, the truth can be faced more fully by the patient. In this phase of coping with disease, people often start fighting and arguing—with their doctors, their relatives, their fate. It is as if they try to overcome the disease by fighting. When they realise this is not possible, it often results in intense feelings of hope and helplessness which can turn into depression. Not everybody is able to finally accept the malignant disease as part of his or her life.

These phases of coping described above were conceptualised by Elisabeth Kübler-Ross after she had interviewed numerous dying patients (Kübler-Ross 2008). Her concept has been adapted by many authors, and at the same time criticised for not being empirically valid. Indeed, these "phases" can be seen in many patients (and their relatives), however, there is no certain order of the "phases" which is why we prefer to call them emotional reactions, that can occur consecutively or simultaneously.

1.2   Denial

Denial allows the patient to keep reality away from the consciousness until he or she is able to deal with it. Clinicians should be aware of the fact that this is a natural process of our psyche to keep our psychological structure alive. At least in the beginning of the cancer trajectory, patients and relatives should get enough time from the medical team until they can refrain from denial. It is not advisable to push them into the truth too fast.

However, continuing denial can be a challenge in oncology, as patients often need to be treated within a short period of time. One should avoid "breaking the denial" by aggressive instructions about the disease and its treatment. This will only result in aggression and anger, be it openly expressed or more silent.

A better way of supporting the patient in getting over his denial is to (a) strengthen his psychosocial resources and (b) avoiding denial in ones own perspective. Health care providers should try to be neutral and not joining the patient in his or her denial. It is often challenging to not do this because it is seductive, especially when treating young patients, to just avoid the idea of pain and potential death. However, if the patient feels that his carers deny his situation he will be even more convinced that his fate is horrible and that he can not deal with it (if not even the "professionals" can deal with it!). This can also make the patient feel totally alone with his fears. So, if the health care provider can accept the patient in his denial and at the same time be prepared to also talk about distressing topics such as the danger of functional impairment, losses and death, it will support the patient to overcome his denial.

> Example:
> My patient was a 40 year old single mother. She received the diagnose ovarial carcinoma 5 years ago and I had been seeing her since then. While she first wanted to see a psychologist to identify psychological causes of her disease with the aim of then changing her life accordingly to be cured from cancer, she was faced with multiple metastases in her entire body. Still, she thought that psychotherapy can cure her and she asked me to help her visualise her blood and cancer cells because she read in a book that this would cure her.
> I saw her emotional suffering and wanted to support her, at the same time I knew that she had a tumour with a poor prognosis, she had multiple metastases, and she was admitted to the palliative medicine ward at our hospital. Her daughter was 15 years old, the patient described her ex-husband as being alcohol dependent, so she did not want her daughter to live with him.
> The patient seemed torn between the hope of cure and the realisation of nearby death, but the truth was too hard to bear so she denied it and seemed to force all others to share this denial with her. Her physician told me about her refusal to find a solution for her daughter, which needed to be resolved since she was facing death.
> During our next session, the patient told me in tears that her parents said to her: "Girl, make sure you get better soon". When she wanted to talk with them about her fears, they both said: "Forget it, you will be better". This obviously did not help her, as she felt utterly alone. In this situation, I decided to openly ask the patient about her feelings regarding death and dying. No one from the team had done this before feeling sorry for the patient and because she seemed to refuse any conversation about it. However, the patient now reacted relieved. We talked about dying, her experiences with death, her ideas about what happens thereafter, and finally about her daughter living without her.
> The patient deceased two weeks later.

This example shows that, although patients often deny, they can at the same time talk about distressing topics if they experience a supporting relationship with someone they trust and who is not in denial himself.

1.3   Co-morbid Mental Health Conditions

At times, psychological distress can be severe for cancer patients, resulting in clinically relevant mental health conditions. Numerous studies have investigated the frequency of these conditions in cancer patients over the past years.

Several meta-analyses and large multi-centre studies have shown that, during the time of cancer diagnosis, about 30 % of the patients suffer from a mental health condition (Mitchell et al. 2011; Singer et al. 2010, 2013a; Vehling et al. 2012). Less is known however about the course of those conditions during the cancer trajectory.

Available evidence suggests that their frequency does not decrease considerably over time (Bringmann et al. 2008).

Known risk factors for mental disorders in cancer patients are pain, high symptom burden, fatigue, mental health problems in the past and disability (Akechi et al. 2004; Rooney et al. 2011; Banks et al. 2010; Agarwal et al. 2010). There are no consistent correlates of depression in cancer patients (Mitchell et al. 2011).

In some studies alcohol dependence was more common in men (Matheson et al. 2012; Dawson 1996; Kessler et al. 1994; Bronisch et al. 1992; Krauß et al. 2007) and in patients with malignancies in the head and neck, oesophagus and liver (Shimazu et al. 2012; Freedman et al. 2007; Hashibe et al. 2007; Kugaya et al. 2000).

Not only does psychiatric co-morbidity represent enhanced distress of the patients calling for specific support from the medical team it also increases the length of hospital stay (Wancata et al. 2001) and negatively affects survival, if not treated adequately (Kissane 2009; Pinquart et al. 2010). It is therefore highly important to identify patients suffering from mental health disorders as soon as possible. Unfortunately, health care providers often fail in identifying these patients (Singer et al. 2011a; Absolom et al. 2011; Fallowfield et al. 2001; Söllner et al. 2001), resulting in severe under-treatment (Singer et al. 2005; Schwarz et al. 2006; Singer et al. 2011b; Oliffe et al. 2008; Stoppe et al. 1999; Werrbach et al. 1987; Wilhelm 2009).

In a large prospective study with cancer patients we found that of those with mental health conditions, 9 % saw a psychotherapist within 3 months of the diagnosis, 19 % after 9 months and 11 % after 15 months. Mental health care use was higher in patients with children ≤ 18 years (odds ratio 3.3) and somatic co-morbidity (odds ratio 2.6) (Singer et al. 2013a). Interestingly, in this study, uptake of mental health care was equal between men and women, in contrast to findings from studies in the general population (Oliffe et al. 2008; Stoppe et al. 1999; Werrbach et al. 1987; Wilhelm 2009). The admission to mental health care did not differ in patients with different educational attainments.

1.4   Potential Positive Impact

During the past decade, increasing interest has been given to potential benefits of the experience of cancer despite it being challenging and often highly distressing, i.e. whether traumatic experiences can lead to emotional growth in patients and relatives (Hungerbuehler et al. 2011; Kahana et al. 2011; Kim et al. 2011; Love et al. 2011; Demirtepe-Saygili et al. 2011; Fromm et al. 1996). Such posttraumatic growth has been defined as positive psychological change experienced as a result of the struggle with highly challenging life circumstances (Calhoun et al. 2000, 2001). It describes the experience of individuals whose development has surpassed what was present before the struggle with the crises occurred, i.e. people feel that they did not simply "go back to life as usual" but that they feel enriched, wiser, grown, etc. after the crisis.

According to Tedeschi and Calhoun (2004), positive changes can be found in five dimensions, representing different types of posttraumatic growth: greater appreciation of life and changed sense of priorities; warmer, more intimate relationships with others; a greater sense of personal strength; recognition of new possibilities of paths for one's life and spiritual development (Tedeschi et al. 2004).

Individuals' experience of posttraumatic growth depends on several predictors. Many facilitating factors have been reported: younger age, female gender, low consumption of alcohol, low levels of pessimism and depression, high life satisfaction, high levels of extraversion, having an active sexual life and receiving counseling (Cormio et al. 2010; Milam 2004; Mols et al. 2009; Paul et al. 2010; Sheikh 2004; Jansen et al. 2011; Barskova et al. 2009). Benefit finding, a concept similar to posttraumatic growth, depends on the amount of time that has passed since stressor onset, the instrument used and the racial composition of the sample (Helgeson et al. 2006).

To date only a few studies have investigated whether or not psychosocial interventions can help to increase posttraumatic growth after traumatic events or serious illness. Especially in cancer patients, evidence is scare. Own research has shown that art therapy once weekly over a period of 22 weeks in the outpatient setting did not increase posttraumatic growth (Singer et al. 2013b). This finding is in accordance with scepticism towards the concept of growth in the context of adversity, including serious illness and towards positive psychology in general (Coyne et al. 2010).

2   Social Impact

Human beings are social beings. We all share our lives with others and are closely related to others, willingly or unwillingly. This implies that a malignant disease not only affects the psychological aspects of ones life but also social relations. Both dimensions are closely intertwined.

Being a part of a society implies a certain status within that society. That status shapes the image one has and increases or decreases the possibilities to exchange goods. In high income countries, social status is usually defined by income, educational attainment and employment, which is why the term preferred by sociologists is "socio-economic position". Each of these three factors defining this position can be changed by a malignant disease.

2.1   Socioeconomic Position

Low socioeconomic position is known to be associated with poor health on the one hand and with less access to healthcare on the other (Williams 2012; Garrido-Cumbrera et al. 2010; Korda et al. 2009; Habicht et al. 2005; Celik et al. 2000; Jenkins et al. 2008; Lorant et al. 2007; Weich et al. 1998, 2001; Singer et al. 2012).

The socioeconomic position may even decrease after a cancer diagnosis, especially in younger patients if they lose their jobs due to cancer-caused disability (Banks et al. 2010). On the other hand, it is also possible that social problems may decrease or even disappear after a cancer diagnosis, for example if a previously unemployed person receives a pension due to disability.

Vocational rehabilitation of cancer patients differs remarkably between countries. For example, while in Scandinavia about 63 % of all patients returned to work after a total laryngectomy (Natvig 1983) and 50 % did so in France (Schraub et al. 1995) only 11 % could return in Spain (Herranz et al. 1999). Predictors of successful return to work are flexible working arrangements, counseling, training and rehabilitation services, younger age, educational attainment, male gender, less physical symptoms and continuity of care (Mehnert 2011).

Similarly, patients' financial burden depends largely on the country's social system and health care insurances. Specific problems are the so-called "out-of-Pocket-health payments". These are expenses the patient has because of the disease and/or its treatment that are not reimbursed by insurance. In the US, breast cancer patients ($n = 156$) who were insured (either by Medicare, Medicaid, or privately) reported that they spent 597 dollars per month for direct medical costs (e.g. stay at a hospital) without reimbursement, 131 dollars for direct non-medical costs (e.g. transport to the hospital, salary for baby sitters etc.) and 727 dollars for indirect costs (e.g. loss of money to do reduced income) (Arozullah et al. 2004). In contrast, we found that, in a group of German cancer patients ($n = 502$), the average amount spent "out-of-pocket" over 3 months was 98 Euros at the time of diagnosis and 30 Euros 15 months after diagnosis (data unpublished). This study however did not tackle indirect costs.

Regarding the course of financial problems, findings are mixed. In a group of German cancer patients at the time of cancer diagnosis ($n = 799$), 41 % reported having financial difficulties due to the disease while this was increased to 52 % half a year after diagnosis (Schwarz et al. 2008). Similar trends were seen in the US (Arozullah et al. 2004) while others found decreasing (Tsunoda et al. 2007; Arndt et al. 2005) or persisting problems (Sullivan et al. 2007).

Financial difficulties can occur not only in the patients but also in the supporters. There are findings showing that especially male support persons and support persons of survivors in active treatment experience increased expenses (Carey et al. 2012).

2.2   Social Relations

Social relations can be a source of great joy and happiness, but also of heavy conflicts and despair. Most patients experience very good social support, especially at the beginning of the cancer treatment trajectory. Family and friends often spend a lot of time and energy to support the patient. If social support is lacking though, it often leads to increased distress (Mehnert et al. 2010).

At times, social support is experienced negatively, especially if relatives or friends are over-protective implying that the patient is not able to care for himself anymore (Bottomley et al. 1997). This should be kept in mind in clinical practice. For example, a breast cancer patient having a husband does not necessarily mean receiving more support. Clinicians should ask patients how they perceive their support and whether they need help with their social life or not.

Another aspect of social relations should be mentioned here: the desire to have children. In younger patients, family planning can be a challenge, especially in patients receiving chemotherapy or anti-hormonal therapy. Doctors should inform them about future possibilities of getting children and about potential alternatives. If patients can not have children any more although they wished to, this is often experienced as a great loss and the psychosocial and medical team should treat that accordingly.

In conclusion, the impact of malignant diseases on social and psychological aspects of patients' and relatives' daily living can be tremendous. Health care professionals should be equipped with the willingness and competence to address these issues and approach patients actively, offering help and support. If patients do not want that help at a given time, it may be wise to offer it later again. Of course, patients should have the freedom to decline psychosocial support from the professionals, however it might be that they decline out of denial or because it is the only thing they can decline during the time of their cancer treatment. For these reasons, it is good to offer support more than once during the illness trajectory.

References

Absolom K, Holch P, Pini S, Hill K, Liu A, Sharpe M, Richardson A, Velikova G (2011) The detection and management of emotional distress in cancer patients: the views of health-care professionals. Psychooncology 20:601–608

Agarwal M, Hamilton JB, Moore CE, Crandell JL (2010) Predictors of Depression Among Older African American Cancer Patients. Cancer Nurs 33:156–163

Akechi T, Okuyama T, Sugawara Y, Nakano T, Shima Y, Uchitomi Y (2004) Major depression, adjustment disorders, and post-traumatic stress disorder in terminally Ill cancer patients: associated and predictive factors. J Clin Oncol 22:1957–1965

Arndt V, Merx H, Stegmaier C, Ziegler H, Brenner H (2005) Persistence of restrictions in quality of life from the first to the third year after diagnosis in women with breast cancer. J Clin Oncol 23:4945–4953

Arozullah AM, Calhoun EA, Wolf M, Finley DK, Fitzner KA, Heckinger EA, Gorby NS, Schumock GT, Bennett CL (2004) The financial burden of cancer: estimates from a study of insured women with breast cancer. J Support Oncol 2:271–278

Banks E, Byles JE, Gibson RE, Rodgers B, Latz IK, Robinson IA, Williamson AB, Jorm LR (2010) Is psychological distress in people living with cancer related to the fact of diagnosis, current treatment or level of disability? Findings from a large Australian study. Med J Aust 193:S62–S67

Barskova T, Oesterreich R (2009) Post-traumatic growth in people living with a serious medical condition and its relations to physical and mental health: a systematic review. Disabil Rehabil 31:1709–1733

Bottomley A, Jones L (1997) Social support and the cancer patient—a need for clarity. Eur J Cancer Care (Engl) 6:72–77

Bringmann H, Singer S, Höckel M, Stolzenburg J-U, Krauß O, Schwarz R (2008) Longitudinal analysis of psychiatric morbidity in cancer patients. Onkologie 31:343–344

Bronisch T, Wittchen HU (1992) Lifetime and 6-month prevalence of abuse and dependence of alcohol in the munich follow-up-study. Eur Arch Psychiatry Clin Neurosci 241:273–282

Calhoun LG, Cann A, Tedeschi RG, McMillan J (2000) A correlational test of the relationship between posttraumatic growth, religion, and cognitive processing. J Trauma Stress 13:521–527

Calhoun LG, Tedeschi RG (2001) Post-traumatic growth: the positive lessons of loss. In: Neimeyer RA (ed) Meaning reconstruction and the experience of loss. American Psychological Association, Washington

Carey M, Paul C, Cameron E, Lynagh M, Hall A, Tzelepis F (2012) Financial and social impact of supporting a haematological cancer survivor. Eur J Cancer Care 21:169–176

Celik Y, Hotchkiss DR (2000) The socio-economic determinants of maternal health care utilization in Turkey. Soc Sci Med 50:1797–1806

Cormio C, Romito F, Montanaro R, Caporusso L, Mazzei A, Misino A, Naglieri E, Mattioli V, Colucci G (2010) Post-traumatic growth in long term cancer survivors. Cancer Treat Rev 36:S112–S112

Coyne JC, Tennen H (2010) Positive psychology in cancer care: bad science, exaggerated claims, and unproven medicine. Ann Behav Med 39:16–26

Dawson D (1996) Gender differences in the risk of alcohol dependence: United States, 1992. Addiction 91:1831–1842

Demirtepe-Saygili D, Bozo O (2011) Perceived social support as a moderator of the relationship between caregiver well-being indicators and psychological symptoms. J Health Psychol 16:1091–1100

Fallowfield L, Ratcliffe D, Jenkins V, Saul J (2001) Psychiatric morbidity and its recognition by doctors in patients with cancer. Br J Cancer 84:1011–1015

Freedman ND, Schatzkin A, Leitzmann MF, Hollenbeck AR, Abnet CC (2007) Alcohol and head and neck cancer risk in a prospective study. Br J Cancer 96:1469–1474

Fromm K, Andrykowski MA, Hunt J (1996) Positive and negative psychosocial sequalae of bone marrow transplantation: implications for quality of life assessment. J Behv Med 19:221–240

Garrido-Cumbrera M, Borrell C, Palencia L, Espelt A, Rodriguez-Sanz M, Pasarin MI, Kunst A (2010) Social class inequalities in the utilization of health care and preventive services in Spain, a country with a national health system. Int J Health Serv 40:525–542

Habicht J, Kunst AE (2005) Social inequalities in health care services utilisation after eight years of health care reforms: a cross-sectional study of Estonia, 1999. Soc Sci Med 60:777–787

Hashibe M, Bofetta P, Janout V, Zaridze D, Shangina O, Mates D, Szeszenia-Dabrowska N, Bencko V, Brennan P (2007) Esophageal cancer in central and eastern Europe: tobacco and alcohol. Int J Cancer 120:1518–1522

Helgeson VS, Reynolds KA, Tomich PL (2006) A meta-analytic review of benefit finding and growth. J Consult Clin Psychol 74:797–816

Herranz J, Gavilan J (1999) Psychosocial adjustment after laryngeal cancer surgery. Ann Otol Rhinol Laryngol 108:990–997

Holland J, Rowland J (1989) Handbook of Psycho-oncology. Oxford University Press, New York

Hungerbuehler I, Vollrath ME, Landolt MA (2011) Posttraumatic growth in mothers and fathers of children with severe illnesses. J Health Psychol 16:1259–1267

Jansen L, Hoffmeister M, Chang-Claude J, Brenner H, Arndt V (2011) Benefit finding and posttraumatic growth in long-term colorectal cancer survivors: prevalence, determinants, and associations with quality of life. Ger Med Sci DOI: 10.3205/11gmds213, URN: urn:nbn:de: 0183-11gmds2131

Jenkins R, Bhugra D, Bebbington P, Brugha T, Farrell M, Coid J, Fryers T, Weich S, Singleton N, Meltzer H (2008) Debt, income and mental disorder in the general population. Psychol Med 38:1485–1493

Kahana B, Kahana E, Deimling G, Sterns S, VanGunten M (2011) Determinants of altered life perspectives among older-adult long-term cancer survivors. Cancer Nurs 34:209–218

Kessler RC, Mcgonagle KA, Zhao SY, Nelson CB, Hughes M, Eshleman S, Wittchen HU, Kendler KS (1994) Lifetime and 12-month prevalence of Dsm-Iii-R psychiatric-disorders in the United-States—results from the national-comorbidity-survey. Arch Gen Psychiatry 51:8–19

Kim Y, Carver CS, Spillers RL, Crammer C, Zhou ES (2011) Individual and dyadic relations between spiritual well-being and quality of life among cancer survivors and their spousal caregivers. Psychooncology 20:762–770

Kissane D (2009) Beyond the psychotherapy and survival debate: the challenge of social disparity, depression and treatment adherence in psychosocial cancer care. Psychooncology 18:1–5

Korda RJ, Banks E, Clements MS, Young AF (2009) Is inequity undermining Australia's 'universal' health care system? Socio-economic inequalities in the use of specialist medical and non-medical ambulatory health care. Aust N Z J Public Health 33:458–465

Krauß O, Ernst J, Kuchenbecker D, Hinz A, Schwarz R (2007) Prädiktoren psychischer störungen bei tumorpatienten: empirische befunde. Psychother Psychosom Med Psychol 57:273–280

Kübler-Ross E (2008) Interviews mit sterbenden. Kreuz, Stuttgart

Kugaya A, Akechi T, Okuyama T, Nakano T, Mikami I, Okamura H, Uchitomi Y (2000) Prevalence, predictive factors, and screening for psychologic distress in patients with newly diagnosed head and neck cancer. Cancer 88:2817–2823

Lorant V, Croux C, Weich S, Deliege D, Mackenbach J, Ansseau M (2007) Depression and socio-economic risk factors: 7-year longitudinal population study. Br J Psychiatry 190:293–298

Love C, Sabiston CM (2011) Exploring the links between physical activity and posttraumatic growth in young adult cancer survivors. Psycho-oncology 20:278–286

Matheson FI, White HL, Moineddin R, Dunn JR, Glazier RH (2012) Drinking in context: the influence of gender and neighbourhood deprivation on alcohol consumption. J Epidemiol Community Health. doi: 10.1136/jech.2010.112441

Mehnert A (2011) Employment and work-related issues in cancer survivors. Crit Rev Oncol Hematol 77:109–130

Mehnert A, Lehmann C, Graefen M, Huland H, Koch U (2010) Depression, anxiety, post-traumatic stress disorder and health-related quality of life and its association with social support in ambulatory prostate cancer patients. Eur J Cancer Care 19:736–745

Milam JE (2004) Posttraumatic growth among HIV/AIDS patients. J Appl Soc Psychol 34:2353–2376

Mitchell AJ, Chan M, Bhatti H, Halton M, Grassi L, Johansen C, Meader N (2011) Prevalence of depression, anxiety, and adjustment disorder in oncological, haematological, and palliative-care settings: a meta-analysis of 94 interview-based studies. Lancet Oncol 12:160–174

Mols F, Vingerhoets AJJM, Coebergh JWW, van de Poll-Franse L (2009) Well-being, posttraumatic growth and benefit finding in long-term breast cancer survivors. Psychol Health 24:583–595

Natvig K (1983) Laryngectomees in Norway. Study no. 4: social, occupational and personal factors related to vocational rehabilitation. J Otolaryngol 12:370–376

Oliffe JL, Phillips MJ (2008) Men, depression and masculinities: a review and recommendations. J Mens Health 5:194–202

Paul MS, Berger R, Berlow N, Rovner-Ferguson H, Figlerski L, Gardner S, Malave AF (2010) Posttraumatic growth and social support in individuals with infertility. Hum Reprod 25:133–141

Pinquart M, Duberstein PR (2010) Depression and cancer mortality: a meta-analysis. Psychol Med 40:1797–1810

Rooney AG, McNamara S, Mackinnon M, Fraser M, Rampling R, Carson A, Grant R (2011) Frequency, clinical associations, and longitudinal course of major depressive disorder in adults with cerebral glioma. J Clin Oncol 29:4307–4312

Schraub S, Bontemps P, Mercier M, Barthod L, Fournier J (1995) Surveillance et rehabilitation des cancers des voies aero-digestives superieures. (Surveillance and rehabilitation of cancers of upper respiratory and digestive tracts). Rev Prat 45:861–864

Schwarz R, Rucki N, Singer S (2006) Onkologisch kranke als patienten der psychotherapeutischen praxis: beitrag zur qualitätserkundung und psychosozialen versorgungslage. Psychotherapeut 51:369–375

Schwarz R, Singer S (2008) Einführung in die psychosoziale onkologie. Ernst Reinhardt Verlag, München

Sheikh AI (2004) Posttraumatic growth in the context of heart disease. J Clin Psychol Med Settings 11:265–273

Shimazu T, Sasazuki S, Wakai K, Tamakoshi A, Tsuji I, Sugawara Y, Matsuo K, Nagata C, Mizoue T, Tanaka K, Inoue M, Tsugane S (2012) Alcohol drinking and primary liver cancer: a pooled analysis of four Japanese cohort studies. Int J Cancer 130:2645–2653

Singer S, Brown A, Einenkel J, Hauss J, Hinz A, Klein A, Papsdorf K, Stolzenburg J-U, Brähler E (2011a) Identifying tumor patients' depression. Support Care Cancer 19:1697–1703

Singer S, Das-Munshi J, Brähler E (2010) Prevalence of mental health conditions in cancer patients in acute care—a meta-analysis. Ann Oncol 21:925–930

Singer S, Ehrensperger C, Briest S, Brown A, Dietz A, Einenkel J, Jonas S, Konnopka A, Papsdorf K, Langanke D, Löbner M, Schiefke F, Stolzenburg J-U, Weimann A, Wirtz H, König HH, Riedel-Heller SG (2013a) Comorbid mental health conditions in cancer patients at working age—prevalence, risk profiles, and care uptake. Psychooncology (accepted)

Singer S, Götze H, Buttstädt M, Ziegler C, Richter R, Brown A, Niederwieser D, Dorst J, Jäkel N, Geue K (2013b) A non-randomized trial of an art therapy intervention for patients with haematological malignancies to support post-traumatic growth. J Health Psychol 18:934–944

Singer S, Herrmann E, Welzel C, Klemm E, Heim M, Schwarz R (2005) Comorbid mental disorders in laryngectomees. Onkologie 28:631–636

Singer S, Hohlfeld S, Müller-Briel D, Dietz A, Brähler E, Schröter K, Lehmann-Laue A (2011b) Psychosoziale versorgung von krebspatienten—versorgungsdichte und—bedarf. Psychotherapeut 56:386–393

Singer S, Lincke T, Gamper E, Schreiber S, Hinz A, Bhaskaran K, Schulte T (2012) Quality of life in patients with thyroid cancer compared with the general population. Thyroid 22:117–124

Söllner W, DeVries A, Steixner E, Lukas P, Sprinzl G, Rumpold G, Maislinger S (2001) How successful are oncologists in identifying patient distress, perceived social support, and need for psychosocial counselling? Br J Cancer 84:179–185

Stoppe G, Sandholzer H, Huppertz C, Duwe H, Staedt J (1999) Gender differences in the recognition of depression in old age. Maturitas 32:205–212

Sullivan PW, Mulani PM, Fishman M, Sleep D (2007) Quality of life findings from a multicenter, multinational, observational study of patients with metastatic hormone-refractory prostate cancer. Qual Life Res 16:571–575

Tedeschi RG, Calhoun LG (2004) Posttraumatic growth: conceptual foundations and empirical evidence. Psychol Inq 15:1–18

Tsunoda A, Nakao K, Hiratsuka K, Tsunoda Y, Kusano M (2007) Prospective analysis of quality of life in the first year after colorectal cancer surgery. Acta Oncol 46:77–82

Vehling S, Koch U, Ladehoff N, Schön G, Wegscheider K, Heckl U, Weis J, Mehnert A (2012) Prävalenz affektiver und angststörungen bei krebs: systematischer literaturreview und metaanalyse. Psychother Psychosom Med Psychol 62:249–258

Wancata J, Benda N, Windhaber J, Nowotny M (2001) Does psychiatric comorbidity increase the length of stay in general hospitals? Gen Hosp Psychiatry 23:8–14

Weich S, Lewis G (1998) Poverty, unemployment, and common mental disorders: population based cohort study. Br Med J 317:115–119

Weich S, Lewis G, Jenkins SP (2001) Income inequality and the prevalence of common mental disorders in Britain. Br J Psychiatry 178:222–227

Werrbach J, Gilbert LA (1987) Men, gender stereotyping, and psychotherapy—therapists perceptions of male clients. Prof Psychol Res Pract 18:562–566

Wilhelm KA (2009) Men and depression. Aust Fam Physician 38:102–105

Williams J (2012) Geographic variations in health care utilization: effects of social capital and self-interest, and implications for US Medicare policy. Socio-Econ Rev 10:317–342

Fear of Progression

Peter Herschbach and Andreas Dinkel

Abstract

Fear of progression (or fear of recurrence) is an appropriate, rational response to the real threat of cancer and cancer treatments. However, elevated levels of fear of progression can become dysfunctional, affecting well-being, quality of life, and social functioning. Research has shown that fear of progression is one of the most frequent distress symptoms of patients with cancer and with other chronic diseases. As a clear consensus concerning clinically relevant states of fear of progression is currently lacking, it is difficult to provide a valid estimate of the rate of cancer patients who clearly suffer from fear of progression. However, recent systematic reviews suggest that probably 50 % of cancer patients experience moderate to severe fear of progression. Furthermore, many patients express unmet needs in dealing with the fear of cancer spreading. These results underline the necessity to provide effective psychological treatments for clinical levels of fear of progression. A few psychosocial interventions for treating fear of progression have been developed so far. Our own, targeted intervention study showed that dysfunctional fear of progression can be effectively treated with a brief group therapy.

P. Herschbach (✉)
Roman-Herzog-Krebszentrum (RHCCC), Klinikum rechts der Isar Technische Universität München, Trogerstraße26, 81675 Munich, Germany
e-mail: p.herschbach@lrz.tum.de

A. Dinkel
Klinik und Poliklinik für Psychosomatische Medizin und Psychotherapie, Klinikum rechts der Isar Technische Universität München, Langerstraße 3, 81675 Munich, Germany
e-mail: a.dinkel@tum.de

U. Goerling (ed.), *Psycho-Oncology*, Recent Results in Cancer Research 197,
DOI: 10.1007/978-3-642-40187-9_2, © Springer-Verlag Berlin Heidelberg 2014

Contents

1   Introduction.. 12
2   Fear of Disease Progression... 13
    2.1   Excursion: Fear of Progression Versus Fear of Recurrence..................... 13
3   Assessment of Fear of Progression... 15
4   Frequency and Correlates of Fear of Progression... 16
    4.1   Prevalence and Course 17
    4.2   Correlates and Consequences.. 17
    4.3   Couple and Family Perspective 19
5   Psychological Treatment Approaches.. 20
    5.1   Clinical Relevance of Dysfunctional Fear of Progression..................... 20
    5.2   The Munich Approach 20
    5.3   Further Treatments 25
6   Conclusion 26
References.. 27

1   Introduction

There is sound evidence today that about 30 % of all cancer patients suffer from some form of mental disease (Mitchell et al. 2011; Singer et al. 2010; Vehling et al. 2012). The most prevalent diagnoses are depression, anxiety, and adjustment disorders.

These diagnoses are based on a thorough assessment of cancer patients, using some kind of structured clinical interview for diagnosing mental disorders. These measures are related to the current psychiatric classification systems, i.e., DSM or ICD, which were primarily developed for the assessment of (more or less) physically healthy patients with psychological problems. However, there are some limitations of the psychiatric model in medical illness, and the criteria of mental disorders might not generally apply to cancer patients. The psychological symptoms of cancer patients, and other medical patients, sometimes do not fit the usual descriptions and the criteria of common mental disorders. As Gurevich et al. (2002, p. 259) noticed, "the personal tragedy of serious medical illness is not necessarily captured within the bounds of psychiatric illness".

In the field of psycho-oncology, one way to resolve this dilemma was to introduce the concept of distress. This is a broadly defined umbrella term that encompasses a wide range of psychological problems, ranging from severe psychopathological symptoms to mild forms of irritation. According to the US-American National Comprehensive Cancer Network Clinical Practice Guideline, distress is "a multi-factorial unpleasant emotional experience of a psychological (cognitive, behavioral, and emotional), social, and/or spiritual nature that may interfere with the ability to cope effectively with cancer, its physical symptoms and its treatment. Distress extends along a continuum, ranging from common normal feelings of vulnerability, sadness, and fears to problems that can become disabling, such as depression, anxiety, panic, social isolation, and existential and spiritual crisis" (see NCCN

Guideline Distress Management 2013). Distress can be measured by self-report, which is one methodological advantage compared to the interviewer-based assessment of mental disorders.

There are plenty of studies that demonstrate the relevance and frequency of various distress symptoms. In our own work, we found that the fear of the cancer spreading was one of the most frequent and important problems of patients. In a sample of 1.721 patients with different cancer diagnoses, about one-third of the patients acknowledged that being afraid of disease progression was a serious or very serious problem to them. Indeed, this was the problem which received the highest severity rating of all problems that were listed in the distress questionnaire (Herschbach et al. 2004).

In the following, we will provide a description and definition of fear of disease progression; report on its prevalence, course, and correlates; and refer to the psychological treatment of clinical levels of fear or progression.

2   Fear of Disease Progression

It is not unusual for physically ill patients to suffer from fears that are related to various aspects of the illness itself. We referred to these kinds of illness-related fears as *fear of progression* (FoP; Dankert et al. 2003).

FoP should be differentiated from the psychiatric concept of anxiety disorders. A central and common characteristic of neurotic anxiety disorders (such as generalized anxiety disorder, panic disorder, and agoraphobia) is that these problems are unreal or irrational. In the context of cancer, however, patients are confronted with real threats; their reactions are neither irrational nor inappropriate. Yet, patients can experience long lasting and exaggerated realistic fears that affect their well-being and quality of life.

Thus, we define FoP as patients' fear that the illness will progress with all its biopsychosocial consequences, or that it will recur. This is a reactive, non-neurotic fear response patients are fully aware of. The fear is based on the personal experience of a life-threatening or incapacitating illness. Like other anxieties, FoP is experienced in emotional, cognitive, behavioral, and physiological qualities. Basically, FoP is an appropriate response to the real threats of diagnosis, treatment, and course of illness. In our view, the level of FoP can range between functional and dysfunctional ends. Elevated levels of FoP that become dysfunctional, i.e., affecting coping, treatment adherence, quality of life, or social functioning, are in need for treatment.

2.1   Excursion: Fear of Progression Versus Fear of Recurrence

The fear of chronically or severely ill patients about the illness getting worse is not a new phenomenon. It seems plausible that this kind of fear is inextricably linked with the experience of severe physical illness. However, it is only in recent years that this kind of fear received more systematic attention in research.

Northouse (1981) provided one of the earliest empirical accounts of cancer patients' fear that the illness might recur. More than a decade later, Lee-Jones et al. (1997) summarized the available, still sparse literature on that topic, and developed a cognitive-behavioral model to explain the exacerbation and maintenance of recurrence fears in cancer patients.

These authors, as well as others, coined the term *fear of recurrence* when speaking of realistic, illness-related fears of cancer patients. So, is there any difference between the two concepts, *fear of progression* and *fear of recurrence*?—Basically, the two concepts are nearly identical.

Our own research on illness-related fears has not been restricted to cancer patients. As our early work revealed, FoP was evident in patients with cancer, rheumatoid arthritis, and diabetes mellitus (Dankert et al. 2003). Furthermore, we discovered that the content of patients' illness-related fears was quite comparable across the studied diseases, with slight nuances concerning predominant fears within each disease group (Dankert et al. 2003). Thus, we conceptualized FoP as a generic concept. To be applicable across a wide range of chronic diseases, we used the term *fear of progression*. This label allows adequately including various diseases with a different disease course, e.g., constantly progressing or remitting-recurring. A further study with more than 800 patients who belonged to 11 disease groups confirmed that FoP is widespread across different diseases (see Fig. 1). Although the disease groups were not directly comparable, owing to differences in the composition of the samples, the results suggested that FoP is a serious concern in rheumatic diseases and some neurologic diseases, too (Berg et al. 2011).

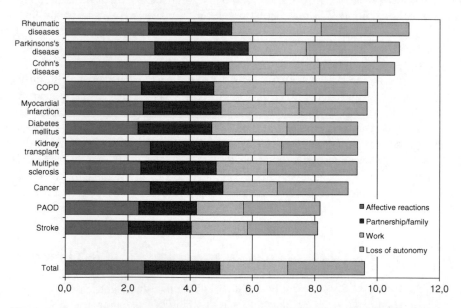

Fig. 1 Fear of progression in different diseases according to subscales and total score of the Fear of Progression Questionnaire (FoP-Q), adapted from Berg et al. (2011) Abbreviations: COPD—chronic obstructive pulmonary disease; PAOD—peripheral artery occlusive disease

The concept of *fear of recurrence* was mainly developed in the field of psycho-oncology. From early days on, it was mainly used to refer to cancer patients in remission, or disease-free cancer patients, who were worried about the cancer coming back (e.g., Northouse 1981). Today, fear of recurrence is defined as "the fear or worry that cancer will return, progress or metastasise" (Crist and Grunveld 2013, p. 978). Another frequently cited definition is usually traced back to the work of Vickberg (2003), although she did not provide this definition verbatim in her paper. It states that fear of recurrence is "the fear that cancer could return or progress in the same place or in another part of the body" (see Koch et al. 2013; Thewes et al. 2012a, b). It is obvious that despite the different labeling, the two constructs *fear of progression* and *fear of recurrence* share relevant defining features and are, basically, comparable. Therefore, we included studies using either one of these two concepts in the writing of this chapter.

3   Assessment of Fear of Progression

As fear of progression has to be distinguished from anxiety disorders, traditional anxiety measures, such as the State-Trait Anxiety Inventory (STAI; Spielberger et al. 1983) or the Beck Anxiety Inventory (Beck and Steer 1993), cannot adequately measure FoP. During the past few years, several self-report measures have been developed that focus specifically on FoP. Recently, Thewes et al. (2012b) provided a systematic review on all current multi-item self-report questionnaires and subscales that assess FoP in cancer patients. They identified 20 multi-item assessment tools, 6 of which being subscales of more comprehensive instruments. Ten measures were classified into the group of brief instruments with 2–10 items. Most of these measures had only limited reliability and validity data available. The remaining four measures fell into the group of longer tools with more than 10 items. These latter measures were judged as reliable and valid. One of these longer self-report measures that had proven reliable and valid is the Fear of Progression Questionnaire (FoP-Q). Actually, the FoP-Q received the highest total quality rating of all instruments, together with the Concerns about Recurrence Scale by Vickberg (see Thewes et al. 2012b).

The FoP-Q is a multidimensional self-reporting questionnaire that was developed in our research group, using samples of patients who were suffering from cancer, rheumatic diseases, and diabetes mellitus (Herschbach et al. 2005). The questionnaire contains 43 items that are rated on a five-point scale, ranging from *never* to *very often*. The items relate to the five dimensions *affective reactions*, *partnership/family issues*, *occupation*, *loss of autonomy*, and *coping with anxiety*. The total score is calculated as the sum of the subscales' mean scores, *excluding* the coping subscale. The questionnaire (total score) has high internal consistency (Cronbach's $\alpha = 0.95$), as well as high test–retest reliability over one week ($r_{tt} = 0.94$) (Herschbach et al. 2005).

Apart from this full version, Mehnert et al. (2006) developed a unidimensional short form, using a sample of breast cancer patients. This abbreviated version, FoP-Q-SF, comprises 12 items pertaining to four of the five subscales (excluding coping). The short form showed adequate reliability ($\alpha = 0.87$); correlational analyses with other psychosocial measures suggested validity. Furthermore, a version for partners of chronically ill patients has been developed and validated, recently, based on the 12-item short form (Zimmermann et al. 2011).

Moreover, the Fear of Progression Questionnaire was translated into two further languages. Shim et al. (2010) provided a Korean version of the full FoP-Q, based on research with a heterogeneous cancer sample. Kwakkenbos et al. (2012) adapted the short form and developed a Dutch version of the FoP-Q-SF, using a sample of patients with systemic sclerosis. Thus, the FoP-Q and the FoP-Q-SF proved to be applicable and useful measures of fear of progression, or fear of cancer recurrence.

Most researchers acknowledge that FoP is an adequate response to the suffering from cancer that, nonetheless, might become dysfunctional. Therefore, it would be highly desirable to identify patients who experience heightened, clinically relevant levels of FoP. However, to date none of the available self-report measures, including FoP-Q and FoP-Q-SF, provides a validated cut-off for the classification of dysfunctional FoP. One reason for this unsatisfying condition is the lack of established external criteria. To date, we do not have a well-established definition of a clinical state of dysfunctional FoP, analogous to the definition of common mental disorders. Consequently, there is no clinical interview to assess and diagnose dysfunctional FoP. Furthermore, it does not seem appropriate to use one of the common anxiety measures as a gold standard, and to conduct sensitivity and specificity analyses of FoP measures in order to establish a clinical cut-off score. Therefore, most researchers who need to define clinical FoP use cut-off scores that are based on statistical considerations, taking into account the distributional characteristics of the measure. Alternatively, cut-off scores are defined on the basis of theoretical considerations.

This shortcoming of the current state of research on FoP has far reaching consequences. As Thewes et al. (2012b) point out, the lack of diagnostic criteria limits comparison between studies, the development of specific interventions, the evaluation of the criterion validity of measures, as well as the development of screening tools indicative of clinical states of FoP.

4   Frequency and Correlates of Fear of Progression

Research on FoP in cancer patients has grown rapidly during the recent years, and the research literature has accumulated. In fact, there are already three systematic reviews on different aspects of FoP in cancer (Crist and Grunveld 2013; Koch et al. 2013; Simard et al. 2013), which underlines the massive interest and efforts put on this topic. Most of this research was conducted with breast cancer patients.

For instance, only 2 of the 17 articles that were included in the systematic review by Koch et al. (2013) included patients who were not diagnosed with breast cancer. In the most comprehensive systematic review, so far, Simard et al. (2013) included 130 papers. The majority of the studies that they had reviewed focused on a specific cancer site, primarily breast cancer (42 studies). However, research also focused, among others, on patients with prostate cancer, ovarian, hematological, or colorectal cancer. Most of the research on FoP was conducted in the United States, but there are also several studies from the UK, Canada, or Germany (see Simard et al. 2013).

In the following, we will briefly refer to the main empirical results on prevalence and correlates of FoP.

4.1   Prevalence and Course

FoP is an appropriate, rational response to the diagnosis of cancer and its treatment. Accordingly, nearly all patients acknowledge feelings of FoP, ranging from very mild upset to severe worries. In Table 1, we present the responses of cancer patients to the items of the Fear of Progression Questionnaire-Short Form (FoP-Q-SF) in women with breast cancer and in a sample with mixed cancer diagnoses. The results show that the vast majority experiences fears and worries. Breast cancer patients, as well as patients with other diagnoses, stated that they are mainly bothered by thoughts about the cancer spreading, worries about severe medical treatments, worries about the next physical examination, and fear of pain.

As there is no clear consensus on clinically elevated FoP, different definitions were applied to define dysfunctional FoP. This limits the comparability of the available data concerning the prevalence of clinical levels of FoP. Prevalence was reported to amount to 47 % in women newly diagnosed with gynecological cancers (Myers et al. 2013), or 56 % in a sample of patients with first-ever cancer diagnosis (Savard and Ivers 2013). Dysfunctional FoP is also high in cancer survivors: 24 % (Mehnert et al. 2009) to 70 % (Thewes et al. 2012a) in breast cancer survivors, 35 % in head and neck cancer survivors (Ghazali et al. 2013), and 31 % in testicular cancer survivors (Skaali et al. 2009).

In their review, Simard et al. (2013) found that, across different cancer sites and assessment strategies, on average 49 % of cancer survivors reported moderate to high degree of FoP, and on average 7 % reported high degree.

Several researchers found that FoP is quite stable over time, with slight decreases in the first months after diagnosis (Savard and Ivers 2013) or during rehabilitation (Mehnert et al. 2013). Simard et al. (2013) report that of 22 longitudinal studies on the course of FoP, eight studies showed that FoP decreased after diagnosis or cancer treatment and then remained stable. The other studies reported no change, or even increase over time. Thus, these results clearly underscore that FoP is a constant companion of cancer patients.

Table 1 Reponses to the items of the Fear of Progression Questionnaire-Short Form (FoP-Q-SF) in two different samples; mean (*M*), standard deviation (SD), and percent of patients (% Positive) experiencing the item at least seldom (scoring at least 2 in the FoP-Q-SF item)

	Breast cancer patients; cancer registry ($N = 1.083$)[a]			Mixed diagnoses; inpatient rehabilitation ($N = 482$)[b]		
	M	SD	% Positive	M	SD	% Positive
I become anxious if I think my disease may progress	2.71	1.12	85.0	3.02	1.06	92.6
I am nervous prior to doctors' appointments or periodic examinations	3.28	1.34	86.9	3.22	1.06	91.1
I am afraid of pain	2.93	1.25	85.0	2.95	1.07	92.1
The thought that I might become less productive at my job disturbs me	2.14	1.39	49.1	2.10	1.31	51.2
When I am anxious, I have physical symptoms, e.g., rapid heartbeat, stomach ache	2.91	1.30	81.4	2.88	1.20	85.9
The possibility of my children contracting my disease disturbs me	2.81	1.54	67.0	2.86	1.42	85.2
It disturbs me that I may have to rely on strangers for activities of daily living	3.08	1.34	84.0	2.88	1.25	85.2
I am worried that at some point in time, because of my illness I will no longer be able to pursue my hobbies	2.38	1.22	69.0	2.46	1.18	75.4
I am afraid of severe medical treatments in the course of my illness	2.80	1.26	82.2	3.08	1.10	91.4
I worry that my medications could damage my body	2.83	1.31	79.7	2.86	1.19	85.0
I worry about what will become of my family if something should happen to me	2.88	1.31	81.0	3.01	1.33	82.0
The thought that I might not be able to work due to my illness disturbs me	2.09	1.32	50.4	2.20	1.24	59.0

Note Item wording of the FoP-Q-SF is taken from Herschbach et al. (2005)
[a]Mehnert et al. (2006)
[b]Herschbach (unpulished data)

4.2 Correlates and Consequences

Research has looked at many potential variables that might correlate and predict FoP. Among potential demographic characteristics, the strongest evidence is for younger age to predict FoP (Crist and Grunveld 2013; Koch et al. 2013; Simard et al. 2013). In contrast to many research results from the field of psychiatry which typically report an association between gender and distress, there is no clear evidence that women experience higher FoP. Similarly, the evidence concerning marital status and FoP is mixed (Crist and Grunveld 2013; Koch et al. 2013;

Simard et al. 2013). Some studies suggest that having children is associated with higher FoP (Mehnert et al. 2009, 2013), but there is also contrasting evidence (Thewes et al. 2012a).

Although some studies reported significant associations among cancer type, disease stage, and treatment-related factors, especially chemotherapy, and FoP, these variables did not predict FoP in most multivariate analyses (Simard et al. 2013). With regard to physical symptoms, there is strong evidence that more frequent or higher number of somatic symptoms are related to higher FoP (Koch et al. 2013; Simard et al. 2013). Thus, the evidence to date suggests that medical and treatment-related factors are of only minor relevance for patients' FoP, except for the presence of somatic complaints.

On the whole, mixed evidence exists for the influence of psychological factors (Koch et al. 2013; Simard et al. 2013). Some results suggest that FoP is higher among cancer patients with high neuroticism, or with low optimism, or with low social support (see Simard et al. 2013), but these results need further replication as they were investigated in only a few studies, so far.

FoP is significantly correlated with distress, depression, anxiety, and traumatic stress symptoms (Simard et al. 2013). These associations are moderately high, showing that FoP is distinct from more general distress or common psychopathological conceptions of emotional disorder.

With regard to the consequences of FoP, there is strong evidence that FoP is related to reduced quality of life and social functioning (Simard et al. 2013). Furthermore, there is some evidence that FoP is related to health care use and health behaviors after cancer diagnosis. Higher FoP was predictive of more unscheduled visits to the general practitioner (Thewes et al. 2012a) and visits to the emergency department (Lebel et al. 2013). Among breast cancer patients, higher FoP was associated with higher frequency of breast self-examination but, interestingly, a lower participation rate in formal medical surveillance, e.g., mammograms or ultrasound. The authors of this study suggest that this behavior pattern is consistent with a cognitive-behavioral model of general health anxiety which postulates that high anxiety is associated with both excessive threat monitoring and avoidance behaviors (Thewes et al. 2012a).

Taken together, despite many research efforts, our knowledge concerning the most potent and relevant predictors of FoP is still limited. The results show that FoP is common and long lasting, and that FoP has a negative impact on patients' lives. However, apart from two or three variables for which there is a quite consistent results pattern, there is mainly mixed evidence regarding the predictive relevance of demographic, illness/treatment-related, and psychological factors.

4.3   Couple and Family Perspective

A very recent trend in research on FoP is the inclusion of partners and family caregivers. One study with relatives of cancer, rheumatoid arthritis, and migraine patients showed that 49 % of the relatives suffered from clinical levels of FoP

(Zimmermann et al. 2012). Studies that included cancer patients as well as their caregivers revealed that FoP was even higher among the family caregivers than in the patient group (Hodges and Humphris 2009; Mellon et al. 2007).

Furthermore, as might be expected, FoP is not only influenced by individual factors, but also by partner effects. One study showed that caregivers' FoP is higher if the patient is in poor physical health (Kim et al. 2012). Another investigation revealed an effect for age; survivors with younger caregivers, as well as caregivers with younger survivors experienced higher levels of FoP (Mellon et al. 2007). Furthermore, one longitudinal study showed that patients' FoP 3 months after diagnosis of head/neck cancer predicted caregivers' FoP at 6 months after diagnosis. No effects of family caregivers' FoP on patients' level were found (Hodges and Humphris 2009).

Thus, these results remind us that cancer is a family affair, and that it is fruitful to adopt a family perspective on FoP. Obviously, this research is only at the beginning, and more research that takes a dyadic, relational approach is needed. Notably, the fact that caregivers express levels of FoP higher than patients should motivate research to develop treatment approaches that also include or are specifically targeted at family caregivers.

5   Psychological Treatment Approaches

5.1   Clinical Relevance of Dysfunctional Fear of Progression

Like other researchers, we conceptualize FoP as an adaptive response that can become dysfunctional. As already shown, the prevalence of FoP is rather high among newly diagnosed cancer patients and among cancer survivors. However, are there any empirical hints that justify the assumption that these are really clinically relevant states?

In our view, there is convincing evidence that FoP in cancer patients can reach levels that are in need of treatment. First, as stated above, FoP is often experienced as the most severe distress symptom (Herschbach et al. 2004). Second, FoP is among the most important concerns cancer patients would like to discuss during their consultation with their oncologist. Research with head and neck cancer patients showed that about 40 % of the patients indicated FoP as their main concern (Kanatas et al. 2013; Rogers et al. 2009). Third, FoP is a main reason for the uptake of psychological treatment. As Salander (2010) reports, anxiety, and worries caused by the disease represented the leading cause for consulting a psychologist. Interestingly, one studied showed that FoP was only seldom the main reason for visiting a general practitioner (Heins et al. 2013). Finally, research has shown that FoP is the most commonly identified unmet psychosocial need of cancer patients, during treatment as well as in the post-treatment phase (Ames et al. 2009; Harrison et al. 2009).

These results corroborate the necessity to identify patients who are suffering from dysfunctional FoP, and to develop and provide appropriate treatments for patients who are experiencing clinically relevant FoP. In the following, we will present, in some detail, a group-based treatment approach that was developed in our research group.

5.2   The Munich Approach

The psychotherapeutic treatment of realistic problems—such as FoP–does not have many predecessors in the professional literature (see Moorey 1996, for an exception). Usually, psychotherapeutic interventions are theoretically related to and developed for neurotic or psychosomatic disorders. Thus, it seemed inevitable to develop a special psychotherapeutic intervention for dysfunctional FoP in physically ill patients.

This new intervention was developed with the guideline that the intervention would be applicable in an inpatient rehabilitation setting. Therefore, it seemed most appropriate to design a brief group-based intervention. The group-based intervention is based on the principles of cognitive-behavioral psychotherapy (CBT). The main general characteristics of this intervention are directiveness and specificity, both aiming at confronting patients with their recurrence fears and supporting patients learning to cope with them. The goal was to learn to manage FoP, in order not to become overwhelmed in daily life. One further treatment goal was to strengthen patients' self-awareness regarding the elicitation and experience of fear. The treatment followed the well-established concepts of cognitive restructuring and worry exposure. Educational elements and homework assignments were also included.

Eventually, this approach comprised four sessions of group psychotherapy (Waadt et al. 2011). Each of the sessions lasted 90 min. The intervention was manualized with regard to structure and content; session topics and interventions were predefined. The session topics are self-awareness and self-assessment, fear exposure, and behavior change and problem-solving. Home-work assignments, diary keeping, and relaxation exercises were used as accompanying interventions.

In the beginning, patients are supported in identifying key personal triggers of FoP, and to describe their subjective experience of FoP. Patients are instructed to differentiate cognitive, behavioral, emotional, and physiological characteristics of their fear response. Patients are educated that experiencing FoP is an adequate response to the real threat of being ill, and that it is necessary to differentiate between functional aspects of FoP and dysfunctional fear levels. The actual cognitive exposure intervention is called "To-Think-the-Fear-to-an-End" (*Zu-Ende-Denken* in German). This intervention resembles the worry exposure, which is used in the treatment of generalized anxiety disorder (Hoyer et al. 2009). Patients are to choose a personally relevant situation that elicits high levels of FoP. In the next step, patients are asked to imagine this situation and to elaborate on all aspects and possible consequences—a task that was usually avoided in daily life, before participation in the group psychotherapy. One such scenario might be loosing one's hair during chemotherapy. An example of a therapeutic dialog with a female patient suffering from the fear of loosing her hair is presented in box 1.

Box 1: Example of cognitive exposure of FoP

Therapist: How will you notice that you start losing your hair?
Patient: I will find hair on my pillow... and in the basin, after hair combing.
Therapist: What will happen in the worst case, what do you think?
Patient: I will also lose my eyebrows.
Therapist: What will be the consequences in your every day life?
Patient: I will feel unfeminine. I will stay at home. I would not go out because people will see that I am a cancer patient. It will be embarrassing for my child, in school when others ask her about her mom.
Therapist: How would you like to react? What do you think would be a competent response, a response you feel well with?
Patient: I'd like to face my cancer, feeling confident, not to hide at home.
Therapist: How could you prepare for this situation?
Patient: I will cut my hair gradually beforehand...I will try wigs and headscarves... I will show myself only to good friends first.

It is assumed that confronting the patient with the possible consequences leads to an increase in perceived control and a reappraisal of the feared consequences. The consequences might get clearer, and the patient might develop helpful ways to deal with the feared consequences. Clearly, the real threat is a real threat is a real threat—however, the cognitive confrontation can demystify diffuse worries to some extent. This helps the patient to find strategies to cope with the actual threats of the disease.

At the end, patients are asked to think about personal changes in coping with FoP as well as changes they would like to implement in their daily lives. Patients are encouraged to choose specific goals that they would like to reach in the next 4 weeks after the end of the group intervention.

As mentioned initially, this group-based intervention was developed for use in inpatient rehabilitation (Waadt et al. 2011). This is a time-limited setting where patients receive multidisciplinary, multimodal therapeutic treatment. It seems reasonable to make necessary adaptations to the treatment protocol, depending on the specific circumstances. For instance, we developed a slightly modified protocol for use with cancer patients who are treated in our outpatient department. Here, we provide a six-session group therapy. We included an introductory session, and we added one more exposure session.

In routine clinical practice, it is essential to inform patients beforehand about the treatment rationale, as this kind of therapy is not suited for all cancer patients. There are patients who feel heavily burdened by clinically elevated FoP but who refrain to join this CBT-based group treatment. Typically, these patients cannot believe that they might tolerate the confrontation with their recurrence fears. These patients will very likely drop out of the therapy if they are not adequately informed about the exposure-based treatment. Obviously, alternative treatments should be offered in this case.

5.2.1 Evaluation

This brief group-based psychotherapeutic treatment was evaluated in a (partially-) randomized controlled trial. As this treatment approach was conceptualized as a generic intervention, applicable to diverse populations, the trial included patients with cancer and patients with rheumatoid arthritis. In the following, we will briefly summarize the trial and the main results, with a special focus on the cancer patients (see Herschbach et al. 2010a, b).

Study Design and Procedure

This was a multicenter, longitudinal (partially-) randomized controlled study. Patients were sampled consecutively during the study, which was conducted in three rehabilitation clinics. Cancer patients were approached in two clinics, arthritis patients came from one clinic. In Germany, admission to inpatient rehabilitation is not necessarily a sign of exacerbation or dramatic worsening of symptoms. Many patients with acute or chronic illness get inpatient rehabilitation treatment in order to re-establish vocational capability, to prevent work disability, or to increase vocational and community participation.

To be eligible for the study, patients had to be at least 18 years old and had to suffer from dysfunctional FoP, i.e., they had to score above a predefined cut-off. The cut-off score for dysfunctional FoP was derived in a separate investigation, conducted before this intervention study, with $N = 130$ arthritis and $N = 150$ cancer inpatients. These patients filled in the short form FoP-Q-SF. In addition, they indicated whether they felt in need of treatment for FoP and would participate in a psychotherapeutic intervention ("yes"/"no"). As there were no external criteria to validate the cut-off score, we followed the conventional strategy of using the median score in a first step. Next, we stratified the sample according to their self-reported treatment need. Thirty-eight percent of the arthritis patients and 36 % of the cancer patients scored above the median and felt in need of treatment. About 10 % in both groups scored above the median and did not express a need for treatment, and about 30 % scored below the median but said they were in need of treatment. These results qualified the median score as a pragmatic cut-off for dysfunctional FoP. The consequence of this approach, which leads to a corresponding rate of treatment need in the two diagnostic groups, was the use of two different median scores. Thus, the predefined FoP-Q-SF cut-off scores for this intervention study were $Md = 38$ for the arthritis patients and $Md = 34$ for the cancer patients.

Patients were randomized into two interventions. Patients in both intervention groups received four sessions of group psychotherapy, each lasting 90 min. The intervention groups were specific to each diagnosis. Groups were designed for a maximum of 10 participants. Both group interventions were conducted as a manualized treatment. The CBT intervention was highly manualized with regard to structure and content. Topics and interventions were predefined, as already described above. The second intervention was a supportive-experiential group intervention (SET). It was manualized with regard to structure, but less prescriptive regarding content. It was based on a client-centered concept and was characterized by nondirectiveness and unspecificity. This intervention aimed at facilitating the expression of personal experiences and emotions, it did not specifically focus on the management of FoP. In each session, the patients decided which topic they would like to discuss. They were supported in reflecting the issues they had selected with regard to FoP. Patients from both intervention groups received two booster phone calls 6 and 9 months after discharge from the clinic. The groups were led by psychotherapists who had at least 3 years of clinical experience and/or who had accomplished or were in the final phase of their therapeutic training.

Originally, the SET intervention was conceptualized as the control condition. However, to exclude that improvement in outcomes was related to overall improvement through the rehabilitation program, a treatment-as-usual control group was sampled after the completion of the intervention phase. These patients did not receive either of the two interventions for reducing FoP. The control group was sampled 1 year after the intervention phase in the same clinics; the same research staff conducted the recruitment using the same eligibility criteria.

Of 457 cancer patients screened, 210 patients were eligible. Of those, 174 (82.8 %) agreed to participate and were assigned to one of the two interventions. In addition, 91 patients were recruited for the control group, resulting in a total sample of $N = 265$ patients. Although patients were not randomly assigned to the control group, our procedure resulted in no relevant systematic differences between the intervention groups and the control group in the measured variables.

FoP was the primary outcome of the study and was assessed using the FoP-Q (full version). Secondary outcomes were anxiety, depression, health-related quality of life, and life satisfaction. Patients from the intervention groups provided data on all outcome measures prior to the initial group therapy session (T1), shortly before discharge from the clinic (T2), 3 months (T3), and 12 months (T4) after discharge. Patients from the control condition only reported on T1, T2, and T4, and they only provided data on the primary outcome FoP.

5.2.2   Results

The mean age of the cancer patients was 53.7 years (SD $= 10.2$), 83 % were women. Not surprisingly, breast cancer was the most frequent diagnosis (58.9 %). 13.1 % of the patients had metastases. The mean illness duration was 19.2 months (SD $= 30.6$).

The results revealed that, compared with treatment-as-usual (TAU), both group therapies were effective in reducing dysfunctional FoP, but only among cancer patients. The effect size were 0.54 for the CBT intervention, 0.50 for the SET intervention, and 0.14 for the TAU group (Herschbach et al. 2010a). As is shown in Fig. 2, the FoP total score significantly declined from pre to post intervention, and continued to decline until 12 months after discharge. In contrast, FoP declined

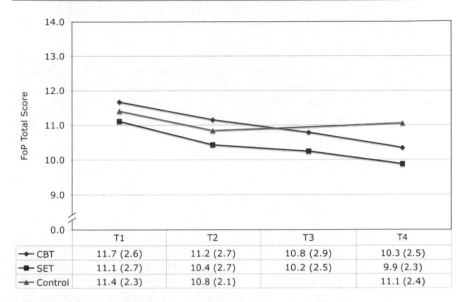

	T1	T2	T3	T4
CBT	11.7 (2.6)	11.2 (2.7)	10.8 (2.9)	10.3 (2.5)
SET	11.1 (2.7)	10.4 (2.7)	10.2 (2.5)	9.9 (2.3)
Control	11.4 (2.3)	10.8 (2.1)		11.1 (2.4)

Fig. 2 Course of fear of progression in different intervention groups during 12 months; total score of the Fear of Progression Questionnaire (FoP-Q) (see Herschbach et al. 2010a) Abbreviations: CBT—cognitive-behavioral group therapy; SET—supportive-experiential group therapy

in the TAU group during inpatient stay, but had reached the initial level after 12 months. There was no effect of intervention type on any secondary outcome.

In a secondary analysis, we aimed to uncover treatment effects beyond the mere reduction of FoP at the group level and, thus, investigated the long-term response to group therapy using the Reliable Change Index (RCI) as response criterion. The results showed that 39.5 % of the cancer patients experienced reliable (though not necessarily clinically significant) improvement 12 months after group therapy. The rate of reliable improvement did not differ according to intervention type. Higher educational level emerged as a significant predictor of reliable change after 12 months (OR 2.53, 95 % CI 1.33–4.81; $p = 0.005$) (Dinkel et al. 2012).

Furthermore, an economic cost-effectiveness evaluation with about 60 patients from the CBT and the SET group, respectively, revealed that group CBT, compared with SET, is cost-effective without the need for additional costs to payers (Sabariego et al. 2011).

In the light of our very brief four session treatment, the effect size as well as the proportion of over one-third of patients who showed a reliable improvement 12 months after the group interventions can be regarded as very promising.

One of the patients who had participated in the CBT intervention provided a vivid account of the helpful experience of this intervention: *"Through 'Thinking-the-Fear-to-an-End' I am not so fearful anymore, I became calmer…The exercise was a 'transformation'. The greatest fear was that I would have to go to a nursing home if the cancer recurs. This is quite unlikely at the moment… However, in case it recurs—I have registered at a nursing home… I do not like to go there but it is an option."*

However, there was no difference in the effectiveness between our newly developed, highly structured CBT intervention, and the less directive SET intervention (except for the economic cost-effectiveness analysis). The reasons are unclear. Yet, there seems to be more than just one single way to reduce dysfunctional FoP in cancer patients.

5.3   Further Treatments

To date, our trial (Dinkel et al. 2012; Herschbach et al. 2010a, b) is the only one that investigated a psychotherapeutic treatment approach that specifically targeted dysfunctional FoP. Apart from this empirical study, there are conceptual publications and trial descriptions on specific interventions for elevated FoP. These protocols describe interventions that are primarily based upon a CBT framework (Butow et al. 2013; Humphris and Ozakinci 2008). Apart from that, there are a few interventions that did not specifically focus on elevated FoP but included it as a secondary outcome. For instance, Lengacher et al. (2009) investigated the effects of mindfulness-based stress reduction (MBSR) for breast cancer survivors. They found that a six-week MBSR program, compared to standard care, reduced FoP from pre to post intervention. However, results on the long-term effects are currently lacking.

Finally, it should be noted that there is one intervention study that focused on couples. This study investigated the effects of a couple-based skills program for women recently diagnosed with breast or gynecological cancer and their partners on FoP and other individual and dyadic outcomes. The effects of the couple-skills intervention were compared to couple cancer education. The results showed that the skills intervention was superior compared to the education intervention in reducing FoP, but only in the short-term. The effect was not maintained over the follow-up period of 16 months (Heinrichs et al. 2012). Thus, this research provides initial evidence for short-term effectiveness of a couple-based intervention in reducing FoP levels in women with cancer. Undoubtedly, as cancer and FoP are also a family affair, more research on the development and evaluation of dyadic and family interventions seems necessary.

6   Conclusion

Many researchers and clinicians have realized that it is necessary and promising to pay special attention to cancer patients' fear of progression. The recent years witnessed a marked increase in research on fear of progression. Several assessment tools were developed, with some instruments reaching high quality ratings. Research revealed some relevant predictors, correlates and consequences of fear of progression. A few psychosocial interventions for treating fear of progression were developed. Results on the efficacy of such interventions are sparse; some trials are under way, some research showed that dysfunctional fear of progression can be effectively treated, as we did show in our own intervention study.

So, what are the main future tasks in research on fear of progression in cancer patients? In our view, the priorities are first, to reach consensus on the definition and measurement of clinical levels of fear of progression; second, to better understand the relevance of illness-related and personal/social factors for dysfunctional fear of progression; and third, to develop, further elaborate and evaluate individual and family-oriented psychological treatments for clinical fear of progression. Accumulating knowledge on these topics should help to provide even better psychosocial care to our patients.

References

Ames J, Crowe M, Colbourne L et al (2009) Patients' supportive care needs beyond the end of cancer treatment: a prospective, longitudinal study. J Clin Oncol 27:6172–6179

Beck AT, Steer RA (1993) Beck anxiety inventory manual. Psychological Corporation, San Antonio

Berg P, Book K, Dinkel A et al (2011) Progredienzangst bei chronischen Erkrankungen [Fear of progression in chronic diseases]. Psychother Psychosom Med Psychol 61:32–37

Butow PN, Bell ML, Smith AB et al (2013) Conquer fear: protocol of a randomised controlled trial of a psychological intervention to reduce fear of cancer recurrence. BMC Cancer 13:201

Crist JV, Grunfeld EA (2013) Factors reported to influence fear of recurrence in cancer patients: a systematic review. Psychooncology 22:978–986

Dankert A, Duran G, Engst-Hastreiter U et al (2003) Progredienzangst bei Patienten mit Tumorerkrankungen, Diabetes mellitus und entzündlich-rheumatischen Erkrankungen [Fear of progression in patients with cancer, diabetes mellitus and chronic arthritis]. Rehabilitation 42:155–163

Dinkel A, Herschbach P, Berg P et al (2012) Determinants of long-term response to group therapy for dysfunctional fear of progression in chronic diseases. Behav Med 38:1–5

Ghazali N, Cadwallader E, Lowe D et al (2013) Fear of recurrence among head and neck cancer survivors: longitudinal trends. Psychooncology 22:807–813

Gurevich M, Devins GM, Rodin GM (2002) Stress response syndromes and cancer: conceptual and assessment issues. Psychosomatics 43:259–281

Harrison JD, Young JM, Price MA et al (2009) What are the unmet supportive care needs of people with cancer? A systematic review. Support Care Cancer 17:1117–1128

Heins MJ, Korevaar JC, Rijken et al (2013) For which health problems do cancer survivors visit their general practitioner? Eur J Cancer 49: 211–218

Heinrichs N, Zimmermann T, Huber B et al (2012) Cancer distress reduction with a couple-based skills training: a randomized controlled trial. Ann Behav Med 43:239–252

Herschbach P, Berg P, Dankert A et al (2005) Fear of progression in chronic diseases. Psychometric properties of the Fear of Progression Questionnaire (FoP-Q). J Psychosom Res 58:505–511

Herschbach P, Berg P, Waadt S et al (2010a) Group psychotherapy of dysfunctional fear of progression in patients with chronic arthritis or cancer. Psychother Psychosom 79:31–38

Herschbach P, Book K, Dinkel A et al (2010b) Evaluation of two group therapies to reduce fear of progression in cancer patients. Support Care Cancer 18:471–479

Herschbach P, Keller M, Knight L et al (2004) Psychological problems of cancer patients: a cancer distress screening with a cancer-specific questionnaire. Br J Cancer 91:504–511

Hodges LJ, Humphris GM (2009) Fear of recurrence and psychological distress in head and neck cancer patients and their carers. Psychooncology 18:841–848

Hoyer J, Beesdo K, Gloster AT et al (2009) Worry exposure versus applied relaxation in the treatment of generalized anxiety disorder. Psychother Psychosom 78:106–115

Humphris G, Ozakinci G (2008) The AFTER intervention: a structured psychological approach to reduce fear of recurrence in patients with head and neck cancer. Br J Health Psychol 13:223–230

Kanatas A, Ghazali N, Lowe D et al (2013) Issues patients would like to discuss at their review consultation: variation by early and late stage oral, oropharyngeal and laryngeal subsites. Eur Arch Otorhinolaryngol 270:1067–1074

Kim Y, Carver CS, Spillers RL et al (2012) Dyadic effects of fear of recurrence on the quality of life of cancer survivors and their caregivers. Qual Life Res 21:517–525

Koch L, Jansen L, Brenner H et al (2013) Fear of recurrence and disease progression in long-term (≥ 5 years) cancer survivors—a systematic review of quantitative studies. Psychooncology 22:1–11

Kwakkenbos L, van den Hoogen FHJ, Custers J et al (2012) Validity of the Fear of Progression Questionnaire-Short Form in patients with systemic sclerosis. Arthritis Care Res 64:930–934

Lebel S, Tomei C, Feldstain A et al (2013) Does fear of recurrence predict cancer survivors health care use? Support Care Cancer 21:901–906

Lee-Jones C, Humphris G, Dixon R et al (1997) Fear of cancer recurrence—a literature review and proposed cognitive formulation to explain exacerbation of recurrence fears. Psychoon-cology 6:95–105

Lengacher CA, Johnson-Mallard V, Post-White J et al (2009) Randomized controlled trial of mindfulness-based stress reduction (MBSR) for survivors of breast cancer. Psychooncology 18:1261–1272

Mehnert A, Berg P, Henrich G et al (2009) Fear of cancer progression and cancer-related intrusive cognitions in breast cancer survivors. Psychooncology 18:1273–1280

Mehnert A, Herschbach P, Berg P et al (2006) Progredienzangst bei Brustkrebspatientinnen—Validierung der Kurzform des Progredienzangstfragebogens PA-F-KF [Fear of progression in breast cancer patients—validation of the short form of the fear of progression questionnaire (FoP-Q-SF)]. Z Psychosom Med Psychother 52:274–288

Mehnert A, Koch U, Sundermann C et al (2013) Predictors of fear of recurrence in patients one year after cancer rehabilitation: a prospective study. Acta Oncol. 52:1102–1109

Mellon S, Kershaw TS, Northouse LL et al (2007) A family-based model to predict fear of recurrence for cancer survivors and their caregivers. Psychooncology 16:214–223

Mitchell AJ, Chan M, Bhatti H et al (2011) Prevalence of depression, anxiety, and adjustment disorder in oncological, haematological, and palliative-care settings: a meta-analysis of 94 interview-based studies. Lancet Oncol 12:160–174

Moorey S (1996) When bad things happen to rational people: cognitive therapy in adverse life circumstances. In: Salkovskis PM (ed) Frontiers of Cognitive Therapy. Guilford, New York, pp 450–469

Myers SB, Manne SL, Kissane DW et al (2013) Social-cognitive processes associated with fear of recurrence among women newly diagnosed with gynecological cancers. Gynecol Oncol 128:120–127

NCCN Guideline Distress Management, Version 2.2103. http://www.nccn.org/professionals/physician_gls/pdf/distress.pdf. Accessed 01 June 2013

Northouse LL (1981) Mastectomy patients and the fear of cancer recurrence. Cancer Nurs 4:213–220

Rogers SN, El-Sheikha J, Lowe D (2009) The development of a Patients Concerns Inventory (PCI) to help reveal patients concerns in the head and neck clinic. Oral Oncol 45:555–561

Sabariego C, Brach M, Herschbach P et al (2011) Cost-effectiveness of cognitive-behavioral group therapy of dysfunctional fear of progression in cancer patients. Eur J Health Econ 12:489–497

Salander P (2010) Motives that cancer patients in oncological care have for consulting a psychologist—an empirical study. Psychooncology 19:248–254

Savard J, Ivers H (2013) The evolution of fear of cancer recurrence during the cancer care trajectory and its relationship with cancer characteristics. J Psychosom Res 74:354–360

Shim EJ, Shin YW, Oh DY et al (2010) Increased fear of progression in cancer patients with recurrence. Gen Hosp Psychiatry 32:169–175

Simard S, Thewes B, Humphris G et al (2013) Fear of cancer recurrence in adult cancer survivors: a systematic review of quantitative studies. J Cancer Suriv 7:300–322

Singer S, Das-Munshi J, Brähler E (2010) Prevalence of mental health conditions in cancer patients in acute care—a meta-analysis. Ann Oncol 21:925–930

Skaali T, Fosså SD, Bremnes R et al (2009) Fear of recurrence in long-term testicular cancer survivors. Psychooncology 18:580–588

Spielberger CD, Gorsuch RL, Lushene R et al (1983) Manual for the state-trait anxiety inventory. Consulting Psychologists Press, Palo Alto

Thewes B, Butow P, Bell ML et al (2012a) Fear of cancer recurrence in young women with a history of early-stage breast cancer: a cross-sectional study of prevalence and association with health behaviors. Support Care Cancer 20:2651–2659

Thewes B, Butow P, Zachariae R et al (2012b) Fear of cancer recurrence: a systematic literature review of self-report measures. Psychooncology 21:571–587

Vehling S, Koch U, Ladehoff N et al (2012) Prävalenz affektiver und Angststörungen bei Krebs: Systematischer Literaturreview und Metaanalyse [Prevalence of affective and anxiety disorders in cancer: systematic literature review and meta-analysis]. Psychother Psychosom Med Psychol 62:249–258

Vickberg SMJ (2003) The concerns about recurrence scale (CARS): a systematic measure of women's fears about the possibility of breast cance recurrence. Ann Behav Med 25:16–24

Waadt S, Duran G, Berg P et al (2011) Progredienzangst. Manual zur Behandlung von Zukunftsängsten bei chronisch Kranken [Fear of progression. Treatment manual]. Schattauer, Stuttgart

Zimmermann T, Alsleben M, Heinrichs N (2012) Progredienzangst gesunder Lebenspartner von chronisch erkrankten Patienten [Fear of progression in partners of chronically ill patients]. Psychother Psychosom Med Psychol 62:344–351

Zimmermann T, Herschbach P, Wessarges M et al (2011) Fear of progression in partners of chronically ill patients. Behav Med 37:95–104

Gender Opportunities in Psychosocial Oncology

Matthew Loscalzo and Karen Clark

Abstract

Avoidance of discussions of sex and gender in medicine reflects the larger lingering societal discomfort with any discussion that links potential sex and gender differences with superiority. The data show that there is more intra-sexual then intersexual variation in men and women. When speaking about sex and gender the literature reflects that, on average, there are many differences, and although they are small, that when taken together, the impact may be quite robust. Sex and gender differences are relevant to how individuals, couples, and families experience and cope with serious illness; however, these important and obvious variables are seldom taken into account when counseling seriously ill patients and their families. Cancer is a complex disease that brings into sharp relief the potential alignments and misalignments in the sexes. In this chapter we have attempted to communicate the imperative for and importance of understanding people under stress within the context of sex and gender. Gender-specific medicine is a very young movement for scientific study but one

Sex does matter. It matters in ways that we did not expect. Undoubtedly, it also matters in ways that we have not begun to imagine. Mary-Lou Pardue, IOM 2001, p X

M. Loscalzo (✉)
City of Hope, 1500 East Duarte Road, Main Medical Bldg Suite Y-1, Duarte, CA 91010-3000, USA
e-mail: Mloscalzo@COH.org

K. Clark
City of Hope, 1500 East Duarte Road Main Medical Bldg Suite Y-8, Durate, CA 91010-3000, USA
e-mail: kclark@coh.org

U. Goerling (ed.), *Psycho-Oncology*, Recent Results in Cancer Research 197, DOI: 10.1007/978-3-642-40187-9_3, © Springer-Verlag Berlin Heidelberg 2014

that has great potential to maximize adaptation and mutual respect at a time when men and women are redefining themselves and adapting to new social realities and challenges.

Contents

1 Sex, Gender Health, and Illness in Context.. 32
2 Sex and Gender Matters.. 33
3 Sexual Dimorphisms is Only Part of the Story but an Important Part......................... 34
4 Getting the Sexes Straight.. 35
5 Clinical Challenges and Opportunities within the Context of Cancer.......................... 37
6 Getting Women and Men to Understand Each Other at their Core: Accessing
   Motivations and Leveraging Natural Inclinations.. 39
   6.1 Understanding and Accessing Motivations 40
   6.2 Natural Inclinations 42
7 Sex and Gender in the Real World 43
8 Summary and Future Directions.. 45
References... 46

1 Sex, Gender Health, and Illness in Context

Avoidance of discussions of sex and gender in medicine reflects the larger lingering societal discomfort with any discourse that links potential sex and gender differences with superiority. At the same time, there are few topics that are of more interest to people (scientists, clinicians, educators, and the public) then how sex and gender influence our daily lives. It has been shown and is now widely accepted that women and men are equally intelligent (Halpern 2000) though the underlying neural mechanisms are clearly different and may in fact be added support for the co-evolution of the sexes (Haier et al. 2005). Recognizing the unique adaptations and resulting strengths and contributions of women and men has a particular significance for coping with illness, for the patient and the caregiver (Loscalzo et al. 2010). The data show that there is more intra-sexual then intersexual variation in men and women (IOM 2001). When speaking about sex and gender the literature reflects that, on average, there are many differences, and although they are small, that when taken together, the impact may be quite robust.

The evolving field of gender specific medicine has been growing rapidly and is gaining additional momentum from the larger interest in and ability to personalize medical care. Genomics, age, sex, gender, personality, behavior, education, and environmental factors all relate to health and illness. There are very few things that can be reliably said about men and women without multiple qualifiers. However, men and women are different and these differences go beyond hormones and genetics. There is still the misperception that sex is primarily or solely related to reproductive functions. The highly influential and provocative 2001 Institute of

Medicine Report: "Exploring the Biological Contributions to Human Health: Does Sex Matter?" documented important sex differences that demonstrate the complexity of sex differences that go far beyond the reproductive system alone. These include: sex chromosomes, immune function, symptom manifestation to same diseases, responses to toxins, brain organization, pain prevalence, and response to medications (IOM 2001). Within this reality, sex and gender differences have significant implications for high–risk populations, screening, assessments, diagnosis, therapy, response, and survival.

Given that men and women are by far much more similar then they are different, questions about why there are sex differences at all are as intriguing as they are provocative and are beyond the focus of this chapter (Buss 2011). The prevailing view proposed by Buss and others is from evolutionary psychology and postulates that women and men have had to adapt to different problems (relating to food, habitat, defense, mate selection, social structures, etc.) (Buss 1995). Over many thousands of years the survival advantages resulting from the successful adaptations sculpted the biology and behavior of the most successful humans–our common progenitors. But as with many other human potentials, the behaviors resulting from these adaptations, and associated with one sex more than the other, are highly flexible, with none, other than reproductive functions, being limited solely to either sex. Evolutionary psychology therefore accurately predicts, across many cultures, that the gatherer (more closely associated with women) would have superior spatial location memory and that the hunter (more closely associated with men) would have a keener sense of spatial rotation (Silverman and Peters 2007). That the potential for women and men solving ongoing problems together, but at times in different ways, is as evident as it is exciting from strengths based perspective. The diversity of perceptions, behaviors, and solutions is evident once there is a willingness to perceive, access, activate, and build on these innate human potentials. Needless to say, there are other explanations relating to sex differences but none have the empirical support of evolutionary psychology (Buss and Schmitt 2011). In fact, Vandermassen in her book, *Who is Afraid of Charles Darwin? Debating Feminism and Evolutionary Theory*, attempts to bridge the empirical chasm between feminist sex role perspectives and that of evolutionary psychology and makes a significant contribution to this complex and evolving field (Vandermassen 2005).

2   Sex and Gender Matters

From the moment of conception there is a defined sex. But sex is anything but simple. Exceptions to clearly defined sex status as female or male is more common than most people realize. For example, the prevalence of disorders of sex development (DSD) (also known as intersex, atypical sex, pseudohermaphroditism) is 1 in 4,000 live births and has gained increasing clinical and public attention (Calleja-Agius et al. 2012). Readers with an interest in this area are referred to the Consensus Statement on Management of Intersex Disorders as this topic is beyond the focus of this chapter (Lee et al. 2006). What is important about DSD is that it demonstrates that both sex and gender are complex and multi-determined and must be seen on a continuum that transcends clearly defined boundaries. But for the vast majority of newborns male or female sex is defined by their genetics. Unfortunately, even in some scientific and medical literature the terms sex and gender continue to be used interchangeably. This has lead to confusion. It is generally agreed that the boundaries between sex and gender are unclear but there are standard definitions that take the overlap into consideration and that lead to greater clarity and credible empirical investigation. In essence, *sex* is seen as biologically determined at birth, one time, by XY chromosomes in males and XX chromosomes in women. While *gender* is a social construct that may change over time. The World Health Organization's definitions of sex and gender are relevant to this discussion and provide insight into the territory, a sense of the complexities involved and a practical common language to understand and address the topic. Sex is defined as "…genetic/physiological or biological characteristics of a person which indicates whether one is female or male…" While gender relates to "women's and men's roles and responsibilities that are socially determined" (World Health Organization 1998, p 10). This description of sex and gender naturally leads to the necessity of understanding "…sex and gender as a single system in which social elements act with biological elements to produce the body has important consequences for medical treatment…genes, physiology, and the physical and social environments operate in concert to produce a phenotype" (IOM 2001, p 10). This context is the foundation for all that follows in this chapter.

3 Sexual Dimorphisms is Only Part of the Story but an Important Part

Sex and gender implications for health are most clearly seen at the beginning and end of life. Women out survive men at birth and also live longer by about 6 years. In the United Sates, this finding has been upheld across all of the 12 ethnic groups measured (National Center for Health Statistics 2011). There is now a very large international literature demonstrating the reality, implications, and importance of sexual dimorphisms and gender differences (Buss et al. 2011). For example, even from the time of birth, although more males are born, 120 males die in the first year for every 100 females. In fact, in the perinatal period males suffer higher rates of morbidity than females in: stillbirths, premature birth, congenital malformations, pulmonary hemorrhage, intracranial hemorrhage, respiratory distress, perinatal asphyxia, perinatal infection, cerebral palsy, developmental delay, Sudden Infant Death Syndrome, Attention Deficit Hyperactivity Disorder, and neurobehavioral difficulties (Rosen and Bateman 2004). There can be no question that these early serious challenges have the potential to negatively impact physical, cognitive, and social development. But sex differences are not limited to early life. Later in life there are also significant sex differences in morbidity and mortality. For example, women are more likely than men to suffer from the following serious illnesses: cardiovascular disease, autoimmune disorders, obesity/diabetes, Post Traumatic Stress Disorder, depression, and anorexia nervosa (Becker et al. 2008). While men are more likely to be diagnosed with cancer, dementias, Parkinson's, mental retardation, autism spectrum disorders (including schizophrenia) substance abuse, and addiction.

It is essential to note that that "sex differences exist at the population level, and as such they should not be used for making inferences about a single individual" and that "…sex differences in the brain and behavior refer to average differences between men and women and that differences between individuals within each sex are much greater than the average differences between sexes" (Resnick and Driscoll 2008). Although in some areas the intersex differences may be small taken together they are very important as it relates to clinical care. In the clinical setting, the manifestations of sex and gender are always influenced to varying degrees and at different times by biology, anthropology, psychology, and societal supports and constraints.

Almost all people see themselves as either men or women regardless of sexual preference. That sex and gender differences are relevant to how individuals, couples, and families experience and cope with serious illness would seem to be apparent but these important and obvious variables are seldom taken into account when counseling seriously ill patients and their families. The very complexity of sex and gender and how it plays out in society and is reflected in the clinical setting may be a deterrent as an open topic for discussion. This is unfortunate and may be a lost opportunity for meaningful communication and joint problem-solving that is at the heart of patient and family centered care. Fortunately, there is an increasing openness in science, medicine, and psychology to empirically understand the complexities of sex and gender. There is also an interest in the general public about how men and women have co-evolved and want to better understand each other. In fact, in many ways, the general public has been more open to the reality of sex and gender differences than have some in the academic community.

4   Getting the Sexes Straight

It may seem paradoxical to say that the differences in the sexes are small but still very important in part because these variations change over time and may be most pronounced during extreme situations. But because these differences may be most obvious under stressful conditions, within a gender-sensitive therapeutic context, these variations are most easy to see and to reframe as immediate opportunities for enhanced mutual understanding, personal growth, and decreased interpersonal conflict. It is also essential to note that although across large population's average sex differences may be small, individual differences in couples, families, or culturally defined groups may be quite robust with high levels of time-sensitive malleability. The cancer experience always involves a larger biopsychosocial context than merely the person diagnosed with cancer and this more realistic perspective, when therapeutically managed, is a unique opportunity to build on internal and external resources that may not have been identified, acknowledged, understood, or utilized.

It is hard to talk about sex or gender differences in the abstract and across large groups but in the clinical setting it is much more obvious and easier to identify and to give voice to the perceptual, attitudinal, and behavioral elements that influence how people struggle to emotionally connect with each other at a core atavistic level. For those men and women who are largely in sync in the manner in which they regulate emotions, respond to threat, and adapt to a rapidly changing environments the relationship will be comforting but may be overly restricted in the diversity of their coping repertoire. Their motivation for exploration and change may also be decreased. A tailored program of psychoeducation may be best suited for this group. In the context of a man and woman who manifests different responses and adaptations to challenges that are different but compatible there is the greatest opportunity for a wide range of coping responses and just enough stress to promote openness to growth. A general program of psychoeducation may be best suited for this group. In the extreme group where the woman and man have gender inclinations that have become a foundation for their life-story, their relationships, and a rigid character structure, distress may be high while motivation will be low and psychotherapy will be the intervention of choice. Ultimately, it is the ability of two or more people to emotionally connect that will influence the level of distress experienced but it is not, with the level of data now available, possible to confidently state the quality of healthy adaptation to the cancer experience overall. This is an area of research that needs to be addressed.

Men and women are too complex to compartmentalize. But it would be disingenuous to ignore compelling paradigms that have empirical support and their relevancy to this discussion—how to help women and men to best support each other during a cancer crisis and beyond. The sexes need to be seen on a continuum. The intra and intersexual differences must always be assessed but when helping individuals it is always a one to one interaction. Many women (as compared to men) may naturally manifest inclinations (e.g., circling the wagons, verbally sharing vulnerabilities, and emotional concerns) that can be clearly identified personally, socially, and culturally as feminine. However, there are many women who do not fit this generalization and who will manifest characteristics that have been traditionally thought of as masculine. While many men (as compared to women) may naturally manifest inclinations (e.g., turning inward, ruminating about fixing the problem, and minimizing the danger through humor) that are associated, identified personally, socially and culturally with masculinities, this is not necessarily an accurate reflection of the male reality. As with women, there are many men who do not match with what historically has been considered to be the masculine expectation never mind the societal ideal. Women, who manifest, has been traditionally masculine traits, are women, and men who manifest has historically been seen as feminine traits are men. The diversity and overlap of human adaptations, by sex specifically, to millennia of dangers and opportunities, are an inherent strength that is far greater than either sex in isolation. This is no less true when men and women confront life-threatening disease, together. We will now share some key information about sex and gender and how it affects patients and couples within the setting of coping with cancer and quality of life.

5 Clinical Challenges and Opportunities within the Context of Cancer

Although the data reviewing sex and/or gender as a primary variable in cancer is quite limited there is a body of literature that is highly informative and is worth a brief review. As it relates to psychological distress, women report more psychological distress overall than do men. This information has been confirmed by many international studies using a wide variety of screening instruments and in diverse cancer populations (Hagedoorn et al. 2008; Zabora et al. 2001). There is no convincing data that can answer the question if women simply feel emotions more intensely, or, if overall, men simply experience emotions less intensely than do women. In our clinical experience, however, the strong impression is that both may be true. We are aware of no published reports in any country or culture where men express emotions or vulnerabilities more openly than do women and this is certainly in part influenced by societal norms. In terms of willingness to report vulnerabilities based on gender, women do report more requests for help (Merckaert et al. 2010) and accept more help (Curry et al. 2002). Women tend to report more distress and unmet needs as it relates to emotional concerns while men tend to focus on more physical problems. It should be noted, however, regardless of the sex of the patient and the country studied, caregivers report higher distress than do cancer patients (Matthews 2003; Kim et al. 2007; Baider et al. 2003). Also within the groups of caregivers, women report more emotional distress than do men (Curry et al. 2002). The essential clinical caveat here is that there is great variation and that every individual needs to be assessed carefully. In the clinical setting, sex and gender are seen as potential *inclinations* that open deeper and more meaningful understandings but not *determinations* that reinforce stereotypes and restricts personal options. But ultimately, the evidence is unequivocal that supportive interpersonal relationships matter, both emotionally and physiologically, and for most people, at least some of these key relationships will be with the opposite sex (Zaider and Kissane 2010). Sex and gender matter because both are very powerful influences (seen and unseen) on the quality of interpersonal relationships and social support. Men and women who have been diagnosed with cancer report that their partners play a key role in their ability to cope and to manage the challenges of the cancer experience. It is a given that spouses or partners are a major support to people diagnosed with cancer. In an important study investigating the partner relationship in response to breast cancer,

Pistrang and Barker found that male partner support (high empathy and low withdrawal) plays a pivotal role in the woman's adaptation and psychological well-being (Pistrang and Barker 1995). While Fergus and Gray (2009) reported that even when women had other strong social supports in place this did not compensate for an unsupportive male partner. Significantly, in a large study of caregivers, Kim et al. (2006) reported that female cancer patients felt that their male partners were very supportive when it came to practical tasks but that they did not provide the emotional support that was so important to them. In essence, men were much more comfortable with demanding and ongoing practical and physical tasks than with the emotional components of the experience. This misalignment has significant implications not only for couples but whenever men and women try to support and connect with each other during times of stress or crisis. The interdependence of spouses and partners highlights the struggles of men and women to identify and to meet each other's expectations and the value that they place on the supportive efforts they manifest. In fact, the authors suggest that the focus on deficit psychology and prevalence of distress overall (as a natural and seductive extension of the medical model) has hindered a more complete picture of people affected by serious illness and their capacities to cope and evolve as individuals and as social systems.

In studies of resiliency, emotional growth, and finding benefit in the cancer experience, relationships have been shown to be particularly crucial. For example, Stanton has summarized a number of studies focusing on what led to benefit-finding or emotional growth in cancer patients. The interpersonal realm, specifically enhanced personal relationships and intimacy (social support) were consistently the most endorsed variables across a number of studies (Stanton 2010). Benefit finding and resiliency research is important to psychosocial oncology because it represents a strengths based approach that can be used to tease out the essential elements of best coping practices. It can be argued that the co-evolution of women and men represents a strength-based process in which the two sexes (including the benefits of heterosexual and same sex orientation) have adapted to each other's needs to insure the short-term and long-term survival of the species. However, the skills that were once essential for the physical survival of the human species have dramatically (and quite suddenly in evolutionary time frames) changed from responding to dangers, challenges, and opportunities in the immediate environment (fast limbic reactions) to highly complex social interactions (slower but more complex pre-frontal cortical processes) aimed at emotional regulation, accurate interpretation of social cues, socially acceptable, and effective social interactions and problem-solving (Kahneman 2011). In the stressful clinical setting, it is helpful to the counselor and therapeutic for the patient and their family caregivers to be able to understand and to reflect these multi-level innate resources in the clinical work.

We will now focus on some gender-specific approaches to helping patients and their caregivers to benefit from understanding the importance of focusing on *motivation over behavior interpretation* and *leveraging natural inclinations.*

6   Getting Women and Men to Understand Each Other at their Core: Accessing Motivations and Leveraging Natural Inclinations

Approximately 65 % of women (ages 25–64) now work outside of the home (Bureau of Labor Statistics 2011). Within the context of the demanding workplace, these are primarily competitive rather than the collaborative relationships that have comprised women's relationships for many millennia. This has been a double stressor for women as they no longer can depend on the support and feedback from other women on a consistent basis to manage their stress. This may leave women feeling emotionally unfulfilled, isolated, diluted, and frustrated. Within the context of cancer, women may turn to men to provide the kind of support which they have historically received from their sisters, mothers, grandmothers, aunts, and female friends. Men are seldom equipped to intuitively respond in a helpful way or to comprehend what women need from them. One of the well-documented gender differences found in the literature is the stress response. When under stress, women have been shown to reach out to others and to "tend and befriend," (Taylor et al. 2000) as an initial response to control their sense of danger and fear. Women feel secure in reaching out to others when trying to manage the stress associated to their vulnerability and do not experience any diminution of self-esteem by asking for help. For women, their level of self-efficacy (i.e., confidence that she can be a good caregiver) has been shown to be an indicator of how they manage stress related to chronic illness (Hagedoorn et al. 2002).

For men, who have traditionally gained their sense of purpose and direction in a highly competitive action oriented environments, such as work, recent social demands focusing on high levels of verbal communication, collaborative team work, and sensitivity to their emotional impact on others has created stress and confusion. Within the context of cancer, both as care recipients and caregivers, many men are confronted with demands from their loved ones that do not come naturally to them and leads to a sense of shame and guilt that encourages their natural inclination to withdraw. When men experience stress, there is an innate tendency to react with the fight-or-flight response. When confronted with stressors who are not manageable by immediate action there is a strong inclination to turn inward to access internal resources and for reflection related to problem-solving. Unlike women, men may experience a sense of diminished self-esteem by sharing their vulnerabilities with others. Although women are adept at prospectively sharing their emotional concerns to reduce their immediate sense of threat, it is only in retrospect that men are generally comfortable sharing their fears and concerns with others, once the sense of threat is reduced to manageable levels. The ways in which many women and men manage their vulnerabilities (women seeking emotional connection and men seeking space and time to think) have significant implications within the context of caregiving. Although female care-givers report higher levels of emotional distress, (Hagedoorn et al. 2008) male caregivers may express their distress by becoming rebellious or aggressive, or by smoking and drinking more (Hagedoorn et al. 2002). At first impression, it would appear that the mismatches of women and men in regulating stress are misaligned and maladaptive. For women, reaching out to a variety of others, verbally processing, sharing detailed internal vulnerabilities, and not expecting resolutions or fixes are natural inclinations for managing stress. For men, turning inward, self-reliance, taking action, outcome orientation, and problem resolution are natural inclinations for managing stress. The changing social demands on women and men when confronted with serious life-threatening illness are different than the more predatory obvious and external dangers for which men and women have had to adapt together throughout history. Cancer is a complex disease that brings into sharp relief the potential alignments and misalignments in the sexes.

What is now expected from women and men in the face of serious threat, such as a cancer diagnosis, may be new to both. In essence, the focus of gender-based interventions is the premise that men and women have the capacity to effectively support each other but that these propensities have not been activated at such an advanced social and psychological level until very recently in evolutionary time. A part of the clinical work is to teach women and men to be open to understand the evolution of men and women successfully working together over many thousands of years and then for them to learn how to be open to broadened perceptions and to activate other innate behaviors that may be less familiar. Sex and gender go well beyond committed sexual partners and often include parents, siblings, friends, bosses, and co-workers. Being able to understand potential gender-based responses, and to reframe them to therapeutic benefit, have the potential to reduce confusion, frustration, and isolation while simultaneously creating an environment of mutual understanding, respect and active problem-solving, ultimately coping. It is a given that when people are under stress they are more likely to revert into their habitual behavioral patterns. In essence, they become more like caricatures of themselves. There are some common behaviors that men and women produce in different frequencies that are generalizations (to be at least considered but never assumed) in the clinical setting. Teaching men and women to get beyond the subjective interpretation of behaviors and to reach for and understand the underlying motivations of their partner can be a potent therapeutic exercise in itself.

6.1   Understanding and Accessing Motivations

The truism that *actions speak louder than words* is only helpful if the actions are interpreted accurately and ultimately leads to a deeper understanding of the behaviors of the actor. For example, in general, humor may be used to deflect the emotional intensity of the situation or to minimize the seriousness of the situation. But a partner may easily see the behavior as disrespectful and emotionally distancing. Making assurances that may not be realistic can also result in a serious misalignment or incongruence (lack of understanding of the other's perspective resulting in increased conflict) (Lewis et al. 2006; Ezer et al. 2011). Our experience has shown us that these are tactics more often used by men. In this situation, the woman may feel that the man is not strong enough and may not be able to be counted on to be there for her when she really needs him. Likewise, when a woman feels confident that she "knows" (because she intuitively feels it so intensely) what her partner is experiencing ("I know that you are angry at me".) and shares her perceptions with her already stressed partner, this may be easily experienced by him as a boundary violation (as well as being incorrect). In this situation, again, everyone loses. The man, feeling powerless and frustrated, may retreat further into the very isolation that the woman was trying to avoid in the first place, which results in her feeling even more alone. These are two very common scenarios that occur within the context of coping with cancer because there is an overreliance on subjective interpretations that is endemic to the mental modeling that all people do in their everyday lives to deal with the multitude of repetitive situations that have to be efficiently managed. But being diagnosed with cancer is not a repetitive experience which most people can delegate to a lower level of reflection. The stress of illness and the potential crisis of cancer require a very large investment of higher cortical functions to emotionally regulate, solve complex problems, make meaning of the situation within a life being lived, and to maintain deep committed emotional connections with others.

Understanding the motivations (what the individual was trying to *achieve* in that specific situation) is a skill that women and men can be taught. Rather than interpreting (making educated/intuitive guesses based on other experiences), teaching women and men how to reach for (and listen with an open mind and an open heart), to the stated motivations of the other person can lead to a positive realignment of the relationship and in the individuals. By putting complex emotions, expectations (rational/irrational), and concerns into language that both people can understand leads to deeper and more authentic communication and emotional connections, even if they disagree. The strengths based assumption here is that when a behavior is being repeated, it is serving some purpose (even if only for the primitive release of physical tension). It is the core purpose (the motivation) that is most important. In most cases the behavior is a signpost but not the destination. Here are some examples of actual scripts that men and women have used in our gender counseling sessions, support and problem-solving groups, and psycho-educational workshops to give voice to their partner's motivations:

- When you spend hours on the internet or watching television, I get confused. Can you please teach me how this helps you to cope with this situation? I want to understand so I do not read into things that will make me feel worse. I need your help to understand.
- When you talk about your cancer in detail to people we hardly know it confuses me and makes me uncomfortable. Can you please teach me how this helps you to talk with strangers about our private matters? I want to be supportive. I really need your help to understand what benefit you get out of this. How does this help you?
- When you make jokes about your cancer and dying, it makes it hard for me to understand what you are going through. It also makes the children and me to

feel more distant from you. Can you please teach me how humor helps you? I really want to understand. How does this help you?

- I am confused and I need your help please. You tell me not to come with you to your doctor appointments. But then when I do not go with you, as you ask, you get enraged at me. What are you trying to achieve by giving me these no-win messages. Please teach me what this is like for you? I care about you and I want to know what you are trying to achieve with these different messages.

Given the emotional intensity and complexity of the life-space in which patients and their caregivers find themselves and the psychological, physical, and spiritual investments to be made over extended periods of time, building on existing behaviors and the natural inclinations of the individual has potential for more positive outcomes. We will now discuss how teaching women and men how to leverage their natural inclinations builds on their existing innate strengths and resources.

6.2   Natural Inclinations

In the classic song Professor Higgins sings, "Why Can't a Woman be More Like a Man?" (My Fair Lady, 1964 song by Frederick Loewe &y Alan Jay Lerner), the stage (a theme repeated too many times in multiple media) is set and so is the trap. By the end of the movie, it is the "Professor" who is educated not only about women but also what it means to be a complete man—the emotional and the intellectual are appreciated. Women and men seldom fit into neat categories—they are both intellectual and have rich emotional lives. In fact, in many parts of the western world, women are now going to colleges and are getting advanced degrees in larger numbers than are men (Aliprantis et al. 2011). The impact of these imminent changes is beyond the scope of this discussion but the need to understand the evolving expectations of the genders is not. In most societies around the world dramatic changes are occurring in the roles, opportunities and expectations for women and men. For example, although women are still the primary caregivers for seriously ill family members, men are increasingly taking on the role as primary caregiving role from 25 % in 1987 to 39 % in 2004, (Kim et al. 2006, 2007). Given the larger numbers of women attaining college and advanced degrees and the decrease in men pursuing higher education in job markets requiring highly skilled labor, dramatic role shifts are expected to accelerate. Within the context of these rapid social changes, men and women will have to be highly adaptable in redefining the roles they value and are prepared to assume in this changing environment. Within the context of cancer, we have seen how in the face of serious life-threatening illness men and women can make major changes in their lives, at times, literally overnight.

The perceptions, attitudes, and behaviors to which people naturally gravitate (the default) when sensing danger can be used as a catalyst for expanding the repertoire of adaptive responses. It is helpful to label these behaviors as "natural inclinations" (Legato 2008) which, as a term, may be less judgmental and stigmatizing and can provide a sense of emotional distance and safety that is essential for the therapeutic context. There is also a connection to a much larger group of known and unknown individuals (in this case women and men) who may share traits and behaviors in common. The added benefit of teaching patients and their caregivers about gender-based natural inclinations is that they can quickly and easily see this process in their own lives and this may lead to a greater openness to learn about and accept the perceptions and responses of others. When people do not perceive the fit into gender-based generalizations this can be reframed into the unique adaptability and flexibility of people to manage the many challenges individuals are forced to manage in their lives as an evolved blend across the sexes. That men or women fit into the generalizations is not important. What is important is that they see their lives as connected to the many courageous and adaptable generations who have come before them and that they have the benefit of building on this legacy, to help them today.

7   Sex and Gender in the Real World

In our work we have focused on teaching men and women to go beyond their subjective interpretations of the behaviors of their loved ones and to try to learn about the subjective *intentions* or *motivations* of the other person. Statements that create an open and honest discussion of the behaviors being manifested are reframed as conversation openers. For example, men and women are taught to ask about behaviors and to not assume or interpret without giving the other person the benefit of the doubt. For instance, we teach men and women to ask specific questions such as; what are you trying to achieve by doing what you are doing? Such as, telling me not to worry, minimizing my concerns, drinking alcohol, bringing up past hurts, making jokes, withdrawing from me physically and emotionally. The men and women are then encouraged to practice this process in the actual session to insure the fidelity of the process and to be sure that they are actually getting to the intention or motivation of the behavior. It will probably not come as surprise to the reader that learning the intention or motivation of the specific behavior reflexively manifested by the man and woman may seem like novel information to them and can enhance motivation to continue the process independent of their work with the clinician. Table 1 lists examples of direct quotes from participants of our gender-specific programs. While Table 2 lists some

Table 1 Examples of quotes from the gender-specific programs

"…oh, is that why he does that, I never would have guessed…"

"…how can she not know that I love her, I am here…"

"…we have been married for 50 years and we never had a conversation like this…"

"…if I would have known how to talk like this I might still be married…"

"…enough of him sharing his feelings, I want my man back…I have feelings too."

Table 2 Women and men solving problem together

What you can do as a partner that is helpful for the woman in your life:
Reflect before reacting to your partner
Communicate with each other in a way that you will be proud of in the future
Actively encourage the sharing of emotional concerns and fears
Be open to help the woman with her physical post surgery care
Listen to concerns without trying to "fix" or minimize them
Be a good listener by listening twice as much as you speak
Only give reassurances that are firmly based in reality (for e.g. "You can count on me")
Be physically present at all medical appointments even when not asked
Learn about the illness and treatments
Help the woman get through the information she needs to read
Take notes and ask questions at medical appointments
Help the woman get things done when the woman can not
Respect and support the woman's right to make her own decisions
Remember that the woman is still a capable individual
Help the woman share information to others she wants to keep informed
Advocate for the woman if needed (whether with health care providers or other family members)
Offer advice only when specifically requested
Be open to listening to the woman expressing her concerns as long as she needs to
What you can do as a woman to get the best out of your partner or family member:
Reflect before reacting to your partner
Be honest and direct about how you feel, especially about your fears
Avoid testing-be specific about what you want from others
Stay in the present-no past hurts or conflicts
No mind-reading-if confused about the behavior of your partner, ask about their motivation
Avoid proving points-focusing on who is right means that you both lose
Tell your partner when you need for them to just listen or when you are seeking advice
Respect that you and your partner might cope with things differently
Access support from peers and/or professionals when needed
Accept help

examples of the guidelines for the men and women who participate in the gender-specific programs and Table 3 lists clinical implications of gender-specific interventions.

Table 3 Clinical implications of gender-specific interventions

Creating therapeutic environments where women and men can more fully appreciate the others individual natural inclinations while celebrating their unique contributions unrestrained by sex or gender

Transcending gender roles can have multiple benefits

Some sex differences become manifest in extreme circumstances only or at certain time (s) only

Identifying, supporting and building on the foundation of natural inclinations of both sexes

Expanding men's skill repertoire to include those used by women

Expanding women's skill repertoire to include those used by men

Benefitting from the inherent synergies of men and women working together

8 Summary and Future Directions

In this chapter we have attempted to communicate the imperative for and importance of understanding people under stress within the context of sex and gender. Gender-specific medicine is a very young movement for scientific study but one that has great potential to maximize adaptation and mutual respect at a time when men and women are redefining themselves and adapting to new social realities and challenges. Fortunately, women and men have been adapting to serious challenges since the beginning of time–together. Most significantly, men and women have insured to survival of the species by co-evolving. For the first time, women and men can be aware of what was a set of complex unconscious processes to one that is now conscious and intentional and this can lead to an acceleration of creative adaptations and emotional growth.

With this appreciation of gender differences in coping and the reciprocal strengths each gender can provide, future research should focus on interventional studies that focus on getting the best out of each gender. These studies are now absent. Such data is important because of the implications for public health, especially mental health, as the world becomes much more complex, automated, and less personally interactive. There is also a need to gain a better understanding of how sex differences leads to vulnerabilities for some and growth for others. The great biopsychosocial complexity of studying sex and gender (and political sensitivities) that have frustrated scientific exploration now creates many exciting opportunities. Ultimately, sex and gender, if for no other reason is worthy of scientific study because it is the most fascinating of stories and it is a story that is still being written, by people like you.

References

Aliprantis D, Dunne T, Fee K (2011) The growing difference in college attainment between women and men. Federal Reserve Bank of Cleveland. http://www.clevelandfed.org/research/commentary/2011/2011-21.cfm. Accessed 28 Sept 2012

Baider L, Ever-Hadani P, Goldzweig G et al (2003) Is perceived family support a relevant variable in psychological distress? A sample of prostate and breast cancer couples. J Psychos Res 55:453–460

Becker JB, Berkley KJ, Geary N et al (2008) Sex differences in the brain: from genes to behavior. Oxford University Press, New York

Bureau of Labor Statistics (2011) Women in the labor force. Available at http://www.bls.gov/cps/wlf-table1-2011.pdf Accessed 1 Oct 2004

Buss DM (1995) Psychological sex differences: Origins through sexual selection. The Am Psychol 50:164–168

Buss DM (2011) Evolutionary psychology: the new science of the mind, 4th edn. Allyn and Bacon, Needham Heights

Buss DM, Schmitt DP (2011) Evolutionary psychology and feminism. Sex Roles 64:768–787

Calleja-Agius J, Mallia P, Sapiano K et al (2012) A review of the management of intersex Neonatal Netw 31:97–103

Curry C, Cossich T, Matthews JP et al (2002) Uptake of psychosocial referrals in an outpatient cancer setting: improving service accessibility via the referral process. Support Care Cancer 10:549–555

Ezer H, Rigol Chachamovich JL, Chachamovich E (2011) Do men and their wives see it the same way? Congruence within couples during the first year of prostate cancer. Psychooncology 20:155–164

Fergus KD, Gray RE (2009) Relationship vulnerabilities during breast cancer: patient and partner perspectives. Psychooncology 18:1311–1322

Hagedoorn M, Sanderman R, Buunk BP et al (2002) Failing in spousal caregiving: the 'identity-relevant stress' hypothesis to explain sex differences in caregiver distress. Br J Health Psychol 7:481–494

Hagedoorn M, Sanderman R, Bolks HN et al (2008) Distress in couples coping with cancer: a meta-analysis and critical review of role and gender effects. Psychol Bull 134:1–30

Haier JR, Jung RE, Yeo RA et al (2005) The neuroanatomy of general intelligence: sex matters. NeuroImage 25:320–327

Halpern DF (2000) Sex differences in cognitive abilities, 3rd edn. Erlbaum, New Jersey

Institute of Medicine (2001) Exploring the biological contributions of human health: does sex matter?. National Academy Press, Washington, DC

Kahneman D (2011) Thinking fast and slow. Farrar, Straus and Giroux, New York

Kim Y, Loscalzo M, Wellisch D et al (2006) Gender differences in caregiving stress among caregivers of cancer survivors. Psychooncology 15:1086–1092

Kim Y, Baker F, Spillers RL (2007) Cancer caregivers' quality of life: effects of gender, relationship, and appraisal. J Pain Symp Manage 34:294–304

Lee PA, Houk CP, Ahmed FS et al (2006) Consensus statement on management of intersex disorders. Pediatrics 118:488–500

Legato MJ (2008) Why men die first. Palgrave MacMillan, New York

Lewis MA, McBride CM, Pollak KI et al (2006) Understanding health behavior change amnion couples: an interdependence and communal coping approach. Soc Sci Med 62:1369–1380

Loscalzo MJ, Kim Y, Clark K (2010) Gender and Caregiving. In: Holland J (ed) Psycho-oncology 2nd edn. Oxford, New York

Matthews BA (2003) Role and gender differences in cancer-related distress: a comparison of survivor and caregiver self-reports. Oncol Nurs Forum 30:493–499

Merckaert I, Libert Y, Messin S et al (2010) Cancer patients' desire for psychological support: prevalence and implications for screening patients' psychological needs. Psychooncology 19:141–149

National Center for Health Statistics. Health, United States (2012) With Special Feature on Socioeconomic Status and Health. Hyattsville, Maryland

Pistrang N, Barker C (1995) The partner relationship in psychological response to breast cancer. Soc Sci Med 40:789–797

Resnick S, Driscoll I (2008) Sex differences in brain aging and Alzheimer's disorders. In: Becker JB et al (ed) Sex differences in the brain: from genes to behavior. Oxford University Press, New York

Rosen TS, Bateman D (2004) The role of gender in neonatology. In: Legato M (ed) Gender-specific medicine. Elsevier Academic Press, London

Silverman I, Choi J, Peters M (2007) The hunter-gatherer theory of sex differences in spatial abilities: data from 40 countries. Arch Sex Behav 36:261–268

Stanton AL (2010) Positive consequences of the experience of cancer: perceptions of growth and meaning. In: Holland J (ed) Psycho-oncology, 2nd edn. Oxford University Press, New York

Taylor SE, Klein LC, Lewis BP et al (2000) Biobehavioral responses in stress in females: tend-and-befriend, not fight-or-flight. Psychol Rev 107:411–429

Vandermassen G (2005) Whos afraid of charles darwin? Debating feminism and evolutionary theory. Rowman and Littlefield, Maryland

World Health Organization (1998) Gender and Health: Technical Paper. Geneva

Zabora J, Brintzenhofeszoc K, Curbow B et al (2001) The prevalence of psychological distress by cancer site. Psychooncology 10:19–28

Zaider TI, Kissane DW (2010) Psychosocial interventions for couples and families coping with cancer. In: Holland J (ed) Psycho-oncology, 2nd edn. Oxford University Press, New York

Psycho-Oncology: A Patient's View

Patricia Garcia-Prieto

Abstract

Culturally the most important, valued, and less stigmatized part of cancer care is the medical part: The surgeon cutting the tumors out and the oncologist leading the strategic decision-making of the medical treatments available. The least valued and stigmatized part of cancer remains the psychosocial care. This chapter describes—through the eyes of an academic, psychologist, stage IV melanoma patient, and patient advocate—how one patient navigated changing psycho-oncological needs from early stage to stage IV through a whole range of psychological interventions available. Her voice joins that of all cancer patients around the world whom are urgently calling for psycho-oncological care to be fully recognized as a central part of cancer treatment.

P. Garcia-Prieto—Deceased

P. Garcia-Prieto (✉)
Centre Emile Berhneim, Solvay Brussels School of Economics and Management,
Université Libre de Bruxelles, Brussels, Belgium
e-mail: pgarciap@ulb.ac.be

P. Garcia-Prieto
Melanoma Independent Community Advisory Board, European Cancer Patient Coalition,
Brussels, Belgium

U. Goerling (ed.), *Psycho-Oncology*, Recent Results in Cancer Research 197,
DOI: 10.1007/978-3-642-40187-9_4, © Springer-Verlag Berlin Heidelberg 2014

Contents

1 A Disclaimer.. 50
2 Psycho-Oncology?.. 50
3 Cancer as My New Psychology Lab.. 50
4 Psycho-Oncology as a Side Dish.. 52
5 Embodying Cancer: Mindfulness-Based Stress Reduction (MBSR)................ 53
6 Meaning and Posttraumatic Growth.. 55
7 Conclusion.. 56
References... 57

1 A Disclaimer

I need to start with a disclaimer. This chapter represents one patient's view on psycho-oncology. I am a stage IV metastatic melanoma patient, president and founder of the Melanoma Independent Community Advisory Board, a pilot project of the European Cancer Patient Coalition (ECPC, Brussels). I am also a psychologist and an academic living in Brussels. I started writing this chapter 1 week after my latest PET-CT scan showed again continued progressive disease. My objective here is to illustrate how my psycho-oncological needs have greatly varied throughout the different stages—Ib to IVc—and describe how I responded to those needs as a function of the psychosocial care that was available to me in my path.

2 Psycho-Oncology?

Psycho-oncology was suggested to me when the first tears welled up during one of my early diagnosis consults in 2008. After an early stage Ib "caught in time" melanoma I had progressed to a stage IIIc by March 2009. I sat in that small stuffy room while my husband told me it would be fine, and the dermatologists and an intern were telling me they would help me take care of it, while the nurse was changing the dressing on it. Like in a bad B movie time stood still and we all did our best to play according to the scripted roles. The hope we all had was that a psycho-oncologist referral would take care of the emotional distress part, which clearly seemed a separate section of cancer care. It was also the one part of my care that we were all the most uncomfortable with. In retrospect, psycho-oncology was presented as a different chapter—if not a different volume—of my cancer story. I did not know at the time that psycho-oncology was in fact a subspecialty of oncology with its own body of knowledge contributing to cancer care. I now know research in this area addresses both (a) patients' psychological reactions to cancer and (b) the psychosocial and behavioral factors that may lead to cancer (Holland 2001). As a patient I have high expectations about (a); and as a researcher I remain skeptical but curious about (b).

3   Cancer as My New Psychology Lab

I was trained as an experimental social psychologist at the University of Queensland in Australia, and I did a Ph.D. in the area of cognitive appraisal theories of emotion at the University of Geneva in Switzerland. When I became "the patient experiencing emotional distress" because of cancer I must confess I initially amused myself by applying well-known stress theories to myself (especially the model of Lazarus and Folkman 1984). I noted the different appraisals that would drive my new cancer emotional landscape including emotions such as numbing fear, anxiety, sadness and despair, and anger and hostility. In fact my Ph.D. thesis was about how our social identities (group memberships) can affect our appraisals and emotions (Garcia-Prieto 2004). I have often used social identity theory strategies (Tajfel and Turner 1986) to counter social identity-threats. For example by creatively redefining my cancer social identity in counter stereotypical ways, or by bringing attention to my professor dimension and away from the patient dimension during an interaction with a doctor, or by engaging in cancer patient advocacy and activism, just to see what would change in me and others. I just have fun with this. After all, even today the cancer social identity remains highly stigmatized by our society and the discrimination one may experience because of the cancer membership can actually lead to increased levels of stress and damage health even more. In a way, with cancer it feels like you have to pay your bill twice as you have to deal with the cancer and you have to deal with the stigma of cancer! So many of my multiple group identities (being an academic, a psychology professor, trained as an experimentalist, working in an economics and business school, codirector of a research center, etc.) represent a great psycho-social resource on which I draw when I am confronted with any hint of discriminatory behavior due to cancer. Of course, the stereotyping of cancer patients is not just done by others (she is a young mother fighting cancer for her children, she is a terminal patient, she is a difficult patient) but also by ourselves (I am an activist battling tooth and nail to join a trial, or I am a resilient cancer patient, I am cancer patient who believes in euthanasia, etc.). There is enough research on how social identities and all the stereotyping and intergroup-related processes can positively and negatively affect health (Hardwood and Sparks 2003). For me it has become an art form to strategically negotiate my way through the many available cancer social identities.

In response to stressful cancer-related situations I have used both problem-focused coping (navigated my care across the best specialties in five hospitals, researching the potential clinical trials I could access before going for my appointments, enquiring about my health rights as a EU citizen, etc.) and emotion-focused coping (binging on dark Belgian chocolate when I would have thoughts of recurrence, purchasing a very expensive leather jacket right after a "bad" PET-CT scan). Truth be told, in that first year after the diagnosis I naïvely thought I knew enough about the psychological aspects of distress to go at it alone. Until the day came that I physically collapsed on the floor in front of my two young kids, exhausted from the interferon injections, and trying to keep up being an academic, mother, wife, and "know it all of the psychology of cancer" patient. I accepted that I was strong enough to search for my first psycho-oncological consultation.

4   Psycho-Oncology as a Side Dish

Luzia Travado (current treasurer of International Psycho-Oncology Society (IPOS)) has reported that there is a great variation in access to psychological services in oncological centers in Europe: if you look at national cancer plans only 19 countries have psycho-oncological services (Beishom 2011). I live in Brussels and thanks to the work of Prof. Darius Razavi the "tracks" of psycho-oncology in Belgium are well defined. I found a great psycho-oncologist and felt comforted by familiar methodologies set clinical goals and experienced results quickly. I wanted a cognitive-behavioral perspective. I did not want a group therapy, I did not want a psychiatrist. I wanted to feel in control, to know the independent variables, mediators, and dependent variables of "my experiment of one". Part of me believed that the psycho-oncological intervention in combination with a good anticancer diet and attitude (Servan-Schreiber 2007) could actually reduce my chances of relapse. At the very least I hoped it would prevent some sort of posttraumatic stress or depression. I did well for a beginner I guess. I knew the cognitive-behavioral approach was sound and evidence-based, proven to be just as good as antidepressants and I felt it worked at least for a while. I then started finding the relief of "relapse-anxiety" would only last the time between consults, and I did not like the feeling of being dependent on the psychologist and on the occasional low-dose Xanax my oncologist could prescribe. Interestingly, like the rest of my medical team (surgeon, dermatologist, oncologist, and nurses) I too perceived my psychological needs as a separate issue, the side dish or dessert, but clearly not as the sauce of the main course! Now I can look back and say without a doubt: psychosocial issues in cancer are grossly underestimated.

I have never heard of the "distress thermometer" or sixth vital sign around me, and I suspect given the amount of distress I have seen in hospital staff, it is clearly not yet measured among oncologists and nurses, surgeons, etc. It has taken me a long time to integrate that the psycho-oncological needs are not "a separate" part, it was the same "me" that was living with the cancer and responding with distress. How could part of me have surgery, radiotherapy, and injections of low-dose interferon and another part of me sit down and cry in the shower hiding from my kids? But that is exactly how we all proceed with psychosocial needs on an implicit and sometimes explicit level. Culturally, the most important and valued and less stigmatized part of cancer care is the medical part: The surgeon cutting the tumors out, the dermatologist doing skin follow-up, and the oncologist leading the strategic decision-making of medical treatments. The least valued and stigmatized part of cancer remains the psychosocial care, an option only to be activated "if need be", maybe even for those who are not strong enough. Though it seems that in the US the science of psychosocial care in oncology and of caring for the whole patient is evolving (Jacobsen et al. 2012) I have not experienced this myself.

5   Embodying Cancer: Mindfulness-Based Stress Reduction (MBSR)

As per text book I have gone through denial, despair, and anger, graduated to bargaining, depression, and have experienced many different levels of acceptance (Kubler-Ross and Kessler 2005). And though I know the theory, nothing prepared me for what the phases of grief would "feel" like in the body. And that was the turning point for me. I was initially caught up in "thinking" about the thoughts and feelings about living with cancer, and despite autohypnosis and relaxation body techniques I was clearly not embodying my cancer experience. This felt like a bit of a paradox: in the case of metastatic melanoma your body gets "intervened" with a lot through surgery. Being an academic did not help. I thought of that well-known movie "Wit" where Emma Thompson plays a professor with stage IV ovarian cancer and how she succeeds in doing a full dose of an innovative chemotherapy cocktail in a trial. She masters that like any other academic project and gains the admiration of her doctors, and then she dies after a trial well done. I have approached cancer and the thoughts and experiences of the life of a patient with advanced melanoma much like I would have approached an experiment too. But in those early years I was not paying attention to the subject's body.

My first attempts to understand the psychological aspects of embodying the cancer experience lead me again to theories and research I knew. Toward the end of my Ph.D., I had seen research on long-term meditators coming out of the prestigious lab of Richard Davidson at the University of Wisconsin-Madison. Two of my best friends had in fact moved from Geneva to Davidson's lab and were there when the study took place and we had talked about it at the time, so I read anything I could find on mindfulness-based stress reduction (MBSR; Kabat-Zinn 1993) and especially as it is related to cancer (Kabat-Zinn et al. 1998) for a good summary see Carlson and Speca (2010) or Shennan et al. (2010) and the immune system more specifically (Davidson et al. 2003; Carlson et al. 2003). I was impressed.

In September 2009, I was still struggling with being an over-anxious IIIc melanoma patient in fear of relapse. I signed up for an 8 week MBSR course at my local hospital. I practiced and asked no questions. I started to become aware of how I felt in my body while I was doing the cancer follow-up routines (medical visits, blood test, follow-up scans, adjuvant treatment, etc.). I noticed the breathing changes, the tensions, the thoughts that would come and go, and the emotions that would visit me quite often. MBSR gave me a new perspective that allowed me to distinguish the thoughts about the cancer situation from the actual experience in the body of those situations. I was able to see that my awareness of my distress was not distressed; that my awareness about fear was not afraid. Work, family life, my couple, and medical experiences all became a perfect lab to test the utility of this new approach. I amazed others and myself at how good I could be at surfing the waves of cancer and at managing to go deep down when the waves became too rough. But had I yet embodied my experience of cancer? Not really.

While I was out surfing a follow-up scan I experienced my own Hokusai great wave. On December 18, 2009, a few days before I drove down to Switzerland with my little family for Christmas I found out I was stage IV and progressing fast. No treatment existed for stage IV melanoma in Belgium. Subcutaneous tumors were popping up like popcorn over the next weeks while my family was worried about the foie gras and the champagne. For the first time I started looking myself for a clinical trial and when I found out that there was one across the border from Brussels (in Paris) but that my health insurance was denying me the right of cross-border health agreements I experienced the most incredible rage I have ever felt in my life. The appraisals of injustice and of high control driving my rage were the fuel of my first steps in patient advocacy mobilizing local media, lawyers, EU politicians. I won that battle with the support of ECPC and others but the trial I fought for could not include me because my tumor burden was too low. I came back to Brussels with a new sense of despair. All throughout this ordeal I held on to MBSR.

The MBSR methodology was easy to follow and I did not need to adhere to any belief system. It was simple and I embraced the new feeling of autonomy and mastery that MBSR practice gave me compared to classic psycho-oncological sessions where I was much more passive and in demand of guidance. With MBSR the guidance was there "online" as things developed, all that I did was show up for what was already there and through each moment of attention given to breath, bodily sensation, thought, or emotion I experienced a strong sense of mastery. Paradoxically, the more I surrendered to what was already happening (tumors coming out, surgery, change of treatment, side effects) the more I felt this sense of mastery. Saki Santorelli describes this beautifully:

> Inwardly speaking, via meditation practice, mastery is cultivated through attending to thoughts, emotions and physical sensations and events in the field of awareness - by allowing these events to arise, be seen, honoured the way they are, and eventually dissipate or dissolve rather than dominate the mind (Santorelli 2011, p. 209).

I did not necessarily like what I experienced and felt, as I was terrified and angry and anxious, or in pain from the surgeries, but the difference was that this time I turned toward those experiences, which were already there anyways, and did not try to change them. Practicing presence or simply "showing up" for whatever the day threw at me radically changed my quality of life, not just life with cancer, but all of my life. I changed my attitude as a teacher, for better or for worse I changed as a wife, mother, daughter, and colleague. But during this period I recognize now that there was also a lot of bargaining with the cancer. I gave myself authority to engage in large projects and accepted increasing responsibility and accepted academic leadership challenges I would have never taken. I know now that it was a way for me to set future goals that I still needed to achieve before

I was "done". And as if by magic, things got done, and I am still setting future goals. My relationship with psycho-oncology changed. I was still heavily relying on help from a psychiatrist for my couple, which was suffering, and sometimes more than my body, but I relied less and less on psycho-oncological consults.

It was also in early 2010 that I started working with a group of like-minded people in Brussels that includes cancer patients like myself, reliable cancer therapies, Association pour le Development du Mindfulness (ADM); The Université Libre de Bruxelles; Institut Jules Bordet; UZ Brussels; UZ Gent; Institute for Attention and Mindfulness, Sint Elisabeth Ziekenhuis (ZNA), and The Chirec cancer institute and a few private sponsors on a long-term project that aims at better integrating mindfulness into oncology centers in Belgium. This work is ongoing and holds great promise on seeing one-day mindfulness-based interventions become standard part of care in oncology centers, and we hope this also becomes reality for the medical/nursing staff.

6   Meaning and Posttraumatic Growth

As the illness has progressed into a stage IV life-limiting illness, and I continue to navigate through clinical trials to extend survival I must confess classic problem— and emotion-focused coping are not enough. MBSR practice without any meaning or spiritual context is also not enough. I am not religious, nor have I been one to search for the "meaning" of life. Thus, as I reach the end I feel I am starting my spiritual awakening from scratch.

I have started more and more to experience what Susan Folkman (1997) has described as meaning-based coping. She has suggested that positive emotions play an important function in stress, and are related to coping mechanisms that are different from those that regulate distress (Folkman 2008). What is interesting in this perspective is that it seems that the coping mechanisms that decrease the negative emotions might be different than those that increase the positive emotions. She talks about the importance of creating the situations that allow for positive emotion. Indeed I am happier now than I have ever been before, and what is interesting is that I feel a quality and intensity of positive emotions that is totally different from pre-cancer positive emotions. I have indeed experienced that it is possible to experience stress from the stage IV situation yet feel both positive and negative emotions during the stress.

Another concept that describes well what I am experiencing now is posttraumatic growth or PTG (Tedeschi and Calhoun 1995). The main idea is that the experience of a highly stressful or traumatic event such as stage IV diagnosis violates one's basic beliefs about the self and the world and that some type of meaning-making or cognitive processing is activated to rebuild these beliefs and goals, resulting in perceptions that one has grown through the process (Tedeschi and Calhoun 2004). A recent meta-analysis of PTG following cancer or HIV/AIDS patients has shown that PTG is related to better positive mental health and self-reported physical health, and less negative mental health (Sawyer et al. 2010).

I have also recently engaged in a process of rediscovering my whole mind–body-spirit dimension. I can imagine this is not the sort of approach that may be readily available in most oncology centers. Yet for me, living with advanced disease, it is the most groundbreaking. I confess that I do not have all the psychological concepts to describe it in much detail here. But the process involves interacting with a therapist that enables me to embody thoughts and emotions, and to perceive what I will call—for lack of a better term—"my sensitive body". I suspect many people discover this dimension and their sensitive body through yoga, reiki, qi gong, tai chi, music or art therapy, or faith. For me this exploration started with meeting and experiencing a session with Jean Paul Resseguier, a French kinésitherapist who developed this method almost 30 years ago. He was influenced by the phenomenology movement (through authors like Edmund Husserl, Maurice Merleau-Ponty and more recently Francisco Varela) and its understanding of the body not as a machine but as a dynamic "living" body that is constantly in a state of "creative" homeostasis interacting within and outside of the body. The Resseguier method has been applied to many medical conditions in Europe and Brasil—including cancer—and patients systematically report better quality of life and enhanced pain management and reduction of side effects during treatment. Unfortunately there is no published research for cancer patients. The major feature of this method is the creation of an empathic relationship ("nouage empathique" in French) between the therapist and the patient through hand-touch in the moment to moment. Basically, you both "show" up for what is there as it unfolds. Concretely for me as an advanced cancer patient it enables me to silently witness the dynamic and sensitive nature of mind–body–spirit. During a session I may experience online physical readjustments that seems to me to occur outside of my conscious "cognitive pilot". These readjustments may be not only physically felt and observed to the naked eye, but also confirmed via medical imagery (in my case the physical readjustments have been recorded via ultrasound and in one case via PET/CT scans). This work, which I continue with a person trained by him Brigitte Maskens in Brussels, has brought me clearly out of my academic comfort zone and for now I am just purely enjoying the ride.

Personally, I must conclude that the awareness of my own death as inevitable leads me to see the absence of all lived possibilities and to hold on to the present as the only place to be. In the words of Merleau-Ponty "present without a future, or an eternal present, is precisely the definition of death" (1945, p. 388).

7   Conclusion

For us, the patients, psycho-oncology should not be presented as a side dish or separate chapter of cancer treatment to be activated only "if need be". Psycho-oncology IS cancer treatment. If empirical evidence of the impact of psychological intervention on overall survival is hard to demonstrate but it is there (see Andersen et al. 2006), there is ample evidence of its positive effect on quality of life, pain reduction and cancer treatment side-effect management. For patients it is clearly not about just extending overall survival, but about living well the time that we live with cancer. Psycho-oncology holds a central place in each step of the path from diagnosis to recovery, and for those who like me live with advanced disease, all the way to the terminal phases of cancer. This central place needs to be recognized and integrated into existing cancer centers, hospitals and national health systems, and cancer plans. Recent reviews leave us with hope that access to psycho-oncological care being facilitated not only in the US but also around the world, and in great part this is due to better-organized patient advocacy and greater inclusion of the patient view in decision-making and debates (Beishom 2011). This chapter is a clear testimony to this.

References

Andersen BL, Hae-Chung Yang WBF, Golden-Kreutz D, Emery C, Thorton LM, Young DC, Carson III WE (2008) Psychologic intervention improves survival for breast cancer patients a randomized clinical trial. Cancer 113(12):3450–3458

Beishom M (2011) Luzia Travado: improving outcomes for patients by attending their distress. Cancer World, London

Carlson LE, Speca M (2010) Mindfulness-based cancer recovery: a step-by-step MBSR approach to help you cope with treatment and reclaim your life. New Harbinger, Oakland

Carlson LE, Speca M, Patel K, Faris P (2007) One year follow-up of psychological, endocrine, immune, and blood pressure outcomes of mindfulness-based stress reduction (MBSR) in breast and prostate cancer outpatients. Brain Behav Immun 21(8):1038–1049

Davidson R, Kabat-Zinn J, Schumacher J, Rosenkrantz M, Muller D, Santorelli S, Urbanowski F et al (2003) Alterations in brain and immune function produced by mindfulness meditation. Psychosom Med 65:564–570

Folkman S (1997) Positive psychological states and coping with severe stress. Soc Sci Med 45:1207–1221

Folkman S (2008) The case for positive emotions in the stress process. Anxiety Stress Copin 21(1):3–14

Garcia-Prieto P (2004) The influence of social identity on appraisal and emotion. Doctoral dissertation. University of Geneva, Faculty of Psychology and Education Sciences, Switzerland. http://www.unige.ch/cyberdocuments/theses2004/Garcia-PrietoP/meta.html

Hardwook J, Sparks L (2003) Social identity and health: an intergroup communication approach to cancer. Health Comm 15(2):145–159

Jacobsen PB, Holland JC, Steensma DP (2012) Caring for the whole patient: the science of psychosocial care. J Clin Oncol 30(11):1151–1153

Kabat-Zinn J (1993) Mindfulness meditation: health benefits of an ancient buddhist practice. In: Goleman D, Gurin J (eds) Mind/Body medicine, consumer reports books. Yonkers, New York

Kabat-Zinn J, Massion AO, Hebert JR, Rosenbaum E (1998) Meditation. In: Holland J (ed) Textbook of psycho-oncology. Oxford University Press, Oxford, pp 767–779

Kübler-Ross E, Kessler D (2005) On grief and grieving: finding the meaning of grief through the five stages of loss. Scribner, New York

Lazarus RS, Folkman S (1984) Stress, appraisal and coping. Springer, New York

Merleau-Ponty M (1945) Phénoménologie de la perception. Gallimard, Paris

Santorelli S (2011) Enjoy your death: leadership lessons forged in the crucible of organizational death and rebirth infused with mindfulness and mastery. Contemporary Budism 12:199–217

Sawyers A, Ayers S, Field AP (2010) Posttraumatic growth and adjustment among individuals with cancer or HIV/AIDS: a meta-analysis. Clin Psychol Rev 30 (4)436–447

Servan-Schreiber D (2007) Anticancer : Prévenir et lutter grâce à nos défenses naturelles. Éditions Robert Laffont S.A

Shennan C, Payne S, Fenlon D (2010) What is the evidence for the use of mindfulness-based interventions in cancer care? A review. Psycho-Oncol 20(7):681–697

Tajfel H, Turner JC (1986) The social identity theory of intergroup behaviour. In: Worschel, S, Austin W.G (eds.) Psychology of intergroup relations. Nelson Hall, Chicago, pp. 7–24

Tedeschi R, Calhoun L (1995) Trauma and transformation: growing in the aftermath of suffering. Sage Publications, Thousand Oaks

Tedeschi R, Calhoun L (2004) Posttraumatic growth: conceptual foundations and empirical evidence. Psychol Inq 15:1–18

The Oncological Patient in the Palliative Situation

Steffen Eychmueller, Diana Zwahlen and Monica Fliedner

Abstract

Palliative care approaches the patient and his or her suffering with a biopsychosocial-spiritual model. Thus, it is the strength of palliative care to complement the diagnosis driven approach of medical cancer care by a problem and resources-based assessment, participatory care plan, and patient-directed interventions. Interventions need to reflect timely prognosis, target population (the patient, the family carer, the professional), and level of trust and remaining energy. In palliative care the relevance of psycho-oncological aspects in the care of the terminally ill is considerable in the understanding of the overall suffering of patients approaching death and their loved ones and in their care and support. There is little evidence to date in terms of clinical benefit of specific psycho-oncological interventions in the last months or weeks of life, but there is evidence on effects of stress reduction and reduced anxiety if locus of control can stay within the patient as long as possible. One major difficulty in psychosocial research at the end-of-life, however, is defining patient relevant outcomes.

S. Eychmueller (✉) · M. Fliedner
University Center for Palliative Care, Inselspital Bern, Bern, Switzerland
e-mail: steffen.eychmueller@insel.ch

D. Zwahlen
Department of Oncology, University Hospital Basel, Bern, Switzerland

U. Goerling (ed.), *Psycho-Oncology*, Recent Results in Cancer Research 197,
DOI: 10.1007/978-3-642-40187-9_5, © Springer-Verlag Berlin Heidelberg 2014

Contents

1 Introduction 61
2 Assessment 62
    2.1 When 62
    2.2 What 63
3 Care Plan 66
    3.1 Multi-professional Teamwork 66
4 Interventions 67
    4.1 Outcomes and Expectations 68
5 Summary 69
References 69

A Patient's Journey: Mrs. B

Mrs. B. is a 58 years formerly very active and athletic woman whose husband died some years ago from cardiac arrest. We, the palliative care inpatient consult team and the patient, met for the first time on a surgical ward where she was hospitalized for abdominal pain and vomiting both due to progressive cholangiocarcinoma. Unintendedly, she broke out into tears when telling about the recent months: after primary surgery she underwent chemotherapy, and despite experience of fatigue she felt pretty well, continued to play tennis, and meet with friends and family. She did not at all expect her cancer to grow during this treatment, and now she feels dramatically disappointed; not only that her cancer was growing again, but also that she misjudged her body's condition. The sudden change in body condition and the new perspective lead to an overall weakness and break down. The former nurse saw herself for the first time in a new role as a patient, dependent on the help of others and most of all as being a burden for her daughter.

We discussed her preferences ("going home, no additional chemotherapy"), her worries ("becoming a burden for her daughter and the whole issues of dying"), her network at home ("nice home, living on my own, daughter with small children living closed by, son abroad for work"), and potential support needs for the future ("most important, providing psychological support for my daughter"). It was proposed to discuss the issues such as role changes in the family and the fear of being a burden and not being able to support others anymore, respectively, together with the psycho-oncologist.

After referral to the palliative care ward we organized a family conference including "skype-link" to her son. Abdominal pain and vomiting improved through medication, complementary therapy, and nutritional counseling. It was the patient herself who finally lead the family conference based on a structured problem-based prompt sheet ("SENS"-structure, i.e., discussion regarding Symptom management, End-of-life decisions based on individual preferences, Network-organization issues for the future care at home, and Support needs of family carers).

Mrs. B. returned home, stayed for several weeks managing symptoms by herself, with little support by her general practitioner, managing her household with external support twice a week, and—most important—meeting regularly with her daughter and grandchildren. Several sessions with the psycho-oncologist lead to open and honest discussions between mother and daughter about family roles, needs, fears, and finally to a better acceptance of role changes and support. The daughter herself wished for further psychotherapeutic support and was referred to a psychotherapist in private practice.

Three days before Mrs. B. died she returned to our palliative care ward accompanied by her entire family, asking for professional help for these last days, recognizing that no energy was left to survive any longer. She was greatly satisfied to have the opportunity to spend valuable time together with her family, experiencing security through the "net" around her and "the final growth, the completion of her life's symphony" even if the end was far too early.

1   Introduction

"Palliative care" or "palliative situation" is still poorly defined and the concept remains vague. Ellen Fox wrote in 1997 a remarkable editorial in the JAMA highlighting the "predominance of the curative model of medical care," as a "residual problem" (Fox 1997). Mrs. B's last weeks could have been easily filled with several medical interventions, which would have resulted in spending most of her remaining lifetime in the hospital. She was in a "palliative situation" and chose the model of care provided by palliative care. Fox continued: "...on a basic level, the curative model conflicts with the notion of a good death." There is a certain danger to omit individual values and goals and the "tendency to perceive patients in terms of their component parts."

Thus, it is the strength of palliative care to complement the diagnosis driven approach of medical cancer care by a problem-based assessment, participatory care plan, and patient-directed interventions. Consequently, palliative care approaches the patient and his or her suffering with a biopsychosocial-spiritual model. It is the aim of palliative care to give back as much self-control as possible to the patient and to provide support wherever and whoever is needed. The target of such care is less a cell or an organ, but the patient and her or his carers—or by words of Dame Cicely Saunders—the unit of care. Collaboration within the palliative care team and among professionals with different backgrounds is a frequent term when discussing and planning patient care. In palliative care the relevance of psycho-oncological aspects is considerable in the understanding of the overall suffering of patients approaching death and their loved ones and in their care and support. Psycho-oncology and palliative care share the view of seeing the patient as a whole and the suffering not only as a medical problem. Both include in their definitions the psychosocial aspects of somatic illness. Both regard the nonmedical aspects as essential part of suffering. Psycho-oncology and palliative care are both frequently involved in the care of patients with advanced cancer, but there is little evidence about "dosage," best time for involvement and process of interaction of these two fields.

There is a substantial overlap of the two definitions of psycho-oncology and palliative care, a fact that explains potential conflicts but which also how they complement each other in daily clinical care. There may be side effects of palliative care and psycho-oncology that need to be recognized early if used alone or in combination. One is adding distress to the patient and family by an overdose of support and/or insufficient coordination of care. Another is to disregard the patient's own resources even in a clinical situation of weakness and frailty, and to focus—as we do in medicine in general—on deficits rather than strengths and resources. In addition, it is of highest importance to distinguish three levels of interaction and reflection: The patient, the patient's surrounding or family, and finally the professional team.

In 2003, Breitbart edited for the first time the journal "Palliative & Supportive Care," "the first international journal of palliative medicine that focuses on the psychiatric, psychosocial, spiritual, existential, ethical, philosophical, and humanities aspects of palliative care" (Breitbart 2003). In a personal reflection Breitbart (2006) challenges one of the most significant values in palliative care and in psycho-oncology: time. Time is of the essence—for reflection, creating trust, and a relationship, doing "unfinished business," coping, communicating, but also for setting priorities: how would I like to spend my remaining lifetime, with whom and where?

This chapter will discuss and highlight recent advances in palliative care with particular focus on psycho-oncological aspects. The authors attempt to focus on data derived from specific studies in a "palliative care" population (which is still difficult to define!): from assessment to interventions having in mind a common "credo": professionalism in palliative care and psycho-oncology relies on the capability to continuously evaluate if treatment and care allow and give back a certain sense of control to the patient and family, of coherence, as Antonovsky defined, even in a "palliative situation"—and provides space and time for essential issues at the end-of-life.

2   Assessment

2.1   When

Possibly THE major issue in palliative care is late referral. In psycho-oncology and palliative care access to this kind of support and care is still lacking clearly defined "red flags," thus the recognition of needs remains unsystematic.

Today, recognition or "diagnosis" of important psychosocial and spiritual distress and palliative care needs in patients with advanced cancer has been highlighted in several guidelines, e.g., (Network 2003). In clinical practice, however, staffing, scientific recognition, routine screening, and financial reimbursement still pose significant barriers for early integration of palliative care in standard oncology care.

There is growing evidence that early integration of palliative care—several months prior to death—not only reduces distress and improves quality of life, but also decreases health care utilization and lastly costs (Temel et al. 2010, 2011; Zhang et al. 2009). Evidence seems to be sufficient for the American Society for Clinical Oncology (ASCO) to recommend early palliative care as best practice in some cancer diagnoses (Smith et al. 2012).

Late referral to psycho-oncological services too is a major issue in cancer care. Psychological disorders like adjustment disorders, anxiety disorders, or depression, only represent a portion of the reasons why cancer patients and their family members should be offered psycho-oncological care. The more general term, distress, is more appropriate for describing the psychosocial difficulties—whether they fulfill the criteria for a psychiatric disorder or not—experienced by many patients and their family members. Estimates are high regarding the number of patients and family members who do not fulfill the formal criteria for a psychological disorder according to the ICD or DSM but they do suffer from clinically relevant psychosocial distress (Bultz and Carlson 2005; Herschbach and Heusser 2008; Holland 2006).

International guidelines also reflect the urgency to quickly and efficiently identify (according to a predefined cut-off) individuals who may require more intense diagnostic and potentially psycho-oncological care (Holland et al. 2007). The standards for care of patients exhibiting psychosocial distress described by the NCCN are of particular importance in this area (National Comprehensive Cancer Network 2003).

Early diagnosis and referral of patients for psychosocial support are especially important with respect to psycho-oncological care, because comorbid psychiatric and psychosocial symptoms not only complicate treatment, but also negatively impact the quality of life of patients and their family members, adversely affect compliance, and lead to poorer medical treatment results (Colleoni et al. 2000; Faller et al. 1999; Ganz 2008; Parker et al. 2003).

2.2 What

Assessing and documenting complexity are one of the big challenges in palliative and end-of-life care. This is also true for the organization of tasks and responsibilities in an inter-professional care team, but also for financial/reimbursement issues. Comprehensive cancer care is one of the attempts to organize such tasks and responsibilities through a shared care model. One of the challenges in highly complex situations as we encounter them in palliative care can be seen in the fact that medical diagnoses alone may not reflect sufficiently individual problems and suffering.

The MASCC Psychosocial Study Group recently published a conclusive paper on main psychosocial concerns and needs of cancer patients and families throughout all phases of the disease (Surbone et al. 2010). In this document we find a call for action in terms of systematic assessment, training and even a "new paradigm of supportive care that addresses psychosocial issues from diagnosis through treatment and post-treatment phases, up to end-of-life or long-term survivorship,..."

Thus, multidimensional assessment of problems or stressors is regarded as highly relevant in palliative care. For the purpose of providing a problem-based assessment system in palliative care, with symptom assessment as only one part of it, the "SENS"-system has been developed (Eychmuller 2012). Adding the problem-based SENS system as a parallel system to medical diagnosis in clinical practice has provided guidance for planning, prevention, concrete care, and coordination of care not only for the patient but also for the family system around him/her. Expectations and hope can be redirected toward actual goals and daily activities instead of medical procedures with sometimes questionable or unclear outcomes.

Other multidimensional or rather multiple-symptom-assessment systems in palliative care are commonly used in clinical practice but all rely on the patient's cognitive function which can alter dramatically even within days or hours. Based on NCCN Clinical Practice Guidelines for Supportive Care, the Edmonton Symptom Assessment System (ESAS) or single item tools for various symptoms (Butt et al. 2008) can be used. As for other tools a score of 4 or more on such screening instruments signifies at least moderately severe symptoms. Most studies on multi-symptom assessment tools are developed and tested mainly in ambulatory patient populations except ESAS.

It is for this reason that assessment in palliative care must be tailored to the patient's situation. Burden and length of the assessment must be minimized and the type of assessment must be related to concrete implications. This means that assessment instruments should have a screening tool character and serve as a foundation to support or enable further communication not necessarily linked directly to the patient but to family and team about the components of despair and possible resources of support. Going back to our patient example, Mrs. B., her distress at the beginning of the contact with the palliative care professionals was the loss of control and her fear to burden her daughter. Her distress did not correspond to symptoms of depression or anxiety nor was it the pain only which made her suffer most. A sensitive and focused dialog only could reveal needs and potential sources of support.

2.2.1 Depression and Anxiety

In a meta-analysis of studies performed with patients in palliative cancer care, Mitchell et al. (2011) reported interesting data. Stratified for various classification systems (ICD, DSM) as well as for stage of disease, this review did not support previous higher percentages of depression in patients with cancer (depression or adjustment disorder 24.7 %, all types of mood disorder 29.0 %). In addition, the study did not reveal any significant difference between palliative care and non-palliative care settings.

Surprisingly, adjustment disorders or anxiety seemed to be slightly more common in non-palliative patients. This might be explained again by the heterogeneous definition of "palliative situation."

Prevalence of anxiety and its relationship to psychological distress in the "palliative patient" is poorly understood. A recent study in terminally ill cancer patients showed moderately increased symptoms of anxiety in 18.6 % and clinically relevant symptoms in 12.4 % of participants. The levels of anxiety did not differ in outpatients versus palliative care inpatients. The Hospital Anxiety and Depression Scale was used to measure symptoms of anxiety and depression, and was administered along with measures of hopelessness, desire for hastened death (Kolva et al. 2011). Palliative care inpatients reported significantly more symptoms of depression and desire for hastened death. The authors believe that an imminent death may lead to an increase of these symptoms.

Anxiety, however, plays an important if not dominant role in symptom perception and expression especially in pain. It is well known from multiple studies in neuropsychology and -physiology that uncertainty and pain are directly linked (Brown et al. 2008; Yoshida et al. 2013). Clinicians therefore need to explore in depth patients' fears and beliefs together with standard symptom assessment.

2.2.2 Demoralization, Hopelessness, and Wish for Hastened Death

There are many components of despair at the end-of-life. While some patients suffer from depression and anxiety others do not fulfill the criteria for these psychiatric diagnoses but suffer from demoralization and hopelessness or loss of meaning—symptoms and syndromes that cannot be categorized according to psychiatric diagnosis. Kissane et al. (2001) wrote an informative article about the importance of demoralization in palliative care, Nissim et al. (2009) investigated the desire for hastened death and hopelessness and Chochinov et al. (2008) looked at dignity. To be aware of and to assess demoralization and hopelessness and the wish for hastened death might be crucial to support some patients in the palliative situation.

2.2.3 Assessing Quality of Life

WHO (2002) defines quality of life as the predominant outcome of palliative care. In clinical practice, however, evaluation of individual quality of life can be difficult. Patients are often too weak and cognitively unstable to provide reliable answers to quality of life assessment tools or questionnaires. In addition most tools have not been evaluated adequately in this challenging clinical situation (Albers et al. 2010). While acknowledging such limitations, highly individualized quality of life measurement tools such as McGill Quality of Life Questionnaire (Cohen and Mount 2000; Cohen et al. 1997) and more recently the SMiLE—instrument (Fegg et al. 2008) have been specifically developed and tested in patients with far advanced cancer or other diseases. The idea behind both instruments, as an example, is to assess individual domains that may contribute to patient-related quality of life and at the same time to give weight to these domains in regard of actual importance. Results from the studies are encouraging but such an approach seems to be linked to research protocols rather than to daily routine.

Intermezzo: Mrs. B

This patient may not be representative for all patients suffering from advanced cancer. Mrs. B. had a long story of self-effectiveness and a rather high level of need of keeping control of her life. Thus, it is no surprise that during assessing her needs and strengths, it was easy to define her goals and to collaborate actively to give weight and priority to various aspects. She was clear in defining worries in regard to her daughter as priority number 1. She was clear in choosing her preferred place of care (at home) and to assess quantity and quality of her individual care team apart from her daughter. She regained control over her miserable illness in the moment, when medical reasoning was complemented by problem-based assessment and care planning. We might underestimate the effect of activating individual coping mechanisms when switching from medical language and diagnosis to day-to-day problems and related problem solving skills.

3   Care Plan

3.1   Multi-professional Teamwork

With increased complexity of the patient and his or her family's situation and depending on the amount of emotional distress in the system, specialized palliative care, and psycho-oncological interventions are required. Thus, in more complex situations the coordination of interdisciplinary support is essential.

Psycho-oncology and palliative care are both frequently involved in patients with advanced cancer, but there is little evidence about "dosage," best time for involvement and process of interaction of these two domains. "The most successful psycho-oncology, psychosocial and behavioral oncology units have been those able to use this diversity to their advantage by evaluating patients and referring them to the most appropriate resource. They function as truly multidisciplinary organizations, drawing on the knowledge of each to enrich the others, while remaining fully integrated in the patients' total medical care"(Holland 2006). The "team" by itself in consequence may become a healing factor—or if distressed and badly coordinated—a risk factor for the patient and family (Nakazawa et al. 2010).

Intermezzo: Mrs. B

The crucial point in Mrs. B.'s patient journey was the moment of taking over the leadership for her remaining lifetime (Detering et al. 2010). Based on her previous life experiences this shift back to control was the key: it was up to her to organize continuity of care and "her" network at home. It was up to her to decide and anticipate that her place for dying might be NOT at home but on the palliative care ward whenever possible; it was up to her to make active plans for the limited amount of time; it was up to her to make peace with her limited physical function.

And it was finally up to her to discuss with her daughter the need for psychological support including the time of bereavement.

4   Interventions

As recommended by various guidelines (e.g., NCCN) best symptom control, advance care planning, and care of the dying should be an integral part of any intervention near the end-of-life. Training in self-administration of drugs (enteral or subcutaneously) by the patient or a family member plays an important role in any crisis intervention (Shipley and Fairweather 2001). Dealing with fatigue and loss of appetite has been reported repetitively to become an important topic in each oncological consultation—not only for the patient, but also for the family (NICE 2011). But palliative care interventions offer more than just "symptomatology," and there might be a danger to overmedicalize treatment.

Not only medical treatment can be overdosed but psycho-oncological support too must be sensitively tailored to the patient and his or her family's situation and the limitations of the circumstances depending on factors such as time, cognitive functioning, and level of energy. Due to limitations and depending on the risk of acute deterioration, interventions usually should be focused on immediate positive effects on despair and acute stressors. As the EAPC paper (European Association for Palliative Care) (Junger and Payne 2011) puts it *In fact, claims regarding the relevance and effectiveness of psychological support provided to dying patients and their relatives should be made with caution. When defining their own professional role, tasks and responsibilities, psychologists should reflect critically upon the real benefits of their contribution. They should avoid a 'pathologisation' or 'psychologisation' of the normal intrapersonal and interpersonal challenges in the context of physical and existential suffering near the end of life.*

A recent qualitative study gives insight to a better understanding of the factors influencing the readiness of patients to address emotional needs (Baker et al. 2012). Results pointed to the fact that many patients do not openly share their emotional difficulties for a variety of reasons. Almost all patients indicated emotional distress or vulnerability. However, for many it felt important not to address distress. The key reason for not wanting to talk about distress was that emotional and mortal vulnerability appeared to be closely linked and patients expected that talking about distress might increase their experience of vulnerability. The key to understand the attitudes of patients was to look at the stage in the treatment trajectory they were at. Recently diagnosed patients were generally negative about being prompted to address distress. Patients interviewed some time after their diagnosis and completed treatment, were generally positive. The study, however, did not include patients on the palliative care ward.

As mentioned above psychiatric diagnoses such as depression and anxiety might be one indication for psycho-oncological support and counseling. But psycho-oncological support in the palliative patient might also be helpful when the components of despair are differing from specific symptoms of psychiatric disorders—as in our patient example Mrs. B.

The EAPC suggests distinguishing between four levels of psycho-oncological interventions in the palliative situation. 1. Compassionate communications and general psychological support, 2. Psychological techniques such as problem solving, 3. Counseling and specific psychological interventions such as anxiety management, and 4. Specialist psychological interventions such as psychotherapy.

Basis of psycho-oncological support and essential for most terminally ill patients and their families is a sustainable and trustful relationship. The importance of the relationship cannot be underestimated in the palliative situation as most patients have a sense of loss of control and vulnerability. The circumstances often lead to a rapidly intensified relationship between patient and psycho-oncologist as well as the awareness of time limits and approaching death might lead to personal developments that can be supported by general psychological support. These aspects demonstrate how difficult it is to measure how and why patients and families might benefit from psycho-oncological support at the end-of-life. One major difficulty in psychosocial research at the end-of-life however is defining patient relevant outcomes.

Nonetheless there is evidence for specialist psycho-oncological interventions with particular tailoring to terminally ill patients as Breitbart et al. (2010, 2012) showed in a meaning centered group setting. One other promising approach is dignity therapy (Chochinov et al. 2011). These first results for a specific population demonstrate both, feasibility, and clinical benefit, and can be considered as promising strategies for the future.

4.1   Outcomes and Expectations

However, one of the major sources for distress—for patients, but also partners/ family and professional carers—can be found in overoptimistic or unrealistic expectations in any intervention in our world of "doing" and feasibility. Calman (1984) introduced a concept in regard to discuss and tailor patient (and carer) expectations as a central strategy to avoid additional distress. These early results have been studied repctitively, among others by Mack et al. in palliative and psycho-oncological care. The Calman gap concept remains one of the pragmatic approaches for physician/psychologist-patient interaction and highlights the importance of the concept of expectations (Broderick et al. 2011). Physical activity frequently cannot be altered or improved which may be difficult to accept especially for sportive people as in our case report. Therefore, physical activity should be replaced or complemented by psychological, social and/or spiritual activity—a strategy that sometimes may patients feel helpless and lost in to date unknown world. Thus, for any intervention we offer to a severely ill person with low level of energy and short timely prognosis, we should consider potential harm in terms of unrealistic expectations and/or lack of individual coping strategies.

5   Summary

Mrs. B. was not able to tell her family and the professional team about her experiences in the very last days of her life. But she could tell the family and the professional carers how important these last weeks at home surrounded by her family were to her. The family on the other hand told the professional team that the joint care planning, its discussion, and finally all interventions responded not only to her mother's needs and wishes, but also integrated at its best the family—and helped to reduce family distress at least to a manageable amount.

Providing space and security for essential things to happen, and to give back a sense of control even in a situation of weakness and fatigue—such elements seem to be mandatory for the final months of life. In times of cost-effectiveness and evidence-based objective measurements this therapeutic approach may be primarily considered as non-scientific, but evidence from neuropsychology, physiology, and from (randomized) controlled trials in assessment and interventions in psychosocial and even spiritual care increasingly support such strategies. The stress-model and recent advances in brain research may add additional evidence and build the bridge to a more scientific acceptance of a humanistic approach. The whole story seems to be about stress reduction and even "healing" in an otherwise desperate life situation, with "healing" being applied not only to the patient, but also to family carers and professionals (Mount and Kearney 2003). Research may finally turn out to support historic findings as formulated earlier by Paracelsus (1493–1541): "Die beste Arznei für den Menschen ist der Mensch. Der höchste Grad dieser Arznei ist die Liebe. Or: the best drug for humans is a human. The highest degree of this drug is love."

References

Albers G, Echteld MA, de Vet HC, Onwuteaka-Philipsen BD, van der Linden MH, Deliens L (2010) Evaluation of quality-of-life measures for use in palliative care: a systematic review. (Eval Stud Rev) Palliat Med 24(1):17–37. doi: 10.1177/0269216309346593
Baker P, Beesley H, Dinwoodie R, Fletcher I, Ablett J, Holcombe C, Salmon P (2012) You're putting thoughts into my head: a qualitative study of the readiness of patients with breast, lung or prostate cancer to address emotional needs through the first 18 months after diagnosis. Psychooncology. doi:10.1002/pon.3156
Breitbart W (2003) Palliative and supportive care: introducing a new international journal; the "Care" journal of palliative medicine. Palliat Support Care 1(1):1–2
Breitbart W (2006) Waiting. Palliat Support Care 4(3):313–314
Breitbart W, Poppito S, Rosenfeld B, Vickers AJ, Li Y, Abbey J, Cassileth BR (2012) Pilot randomized controlled trial of individual meaning-centered psychotherapy for patients with advanced cancer (Comparative study randomized controlled trial research support, non-US gov't). J Clin Oncol, 30(12):1304–1309. doi: 10.1200/JCO.2011.36.2517
Breitbart W, Rosenfeld B, Gibson C, Pessin H, Poppito S, Nelson C, Olden M (2010) Meaning-centered group psychotherapy for patients with advanced cancer: a pilot randomized controlled trial (Randomized controlled trial research support, NIH, extramural research support, non-US gov't). Psychooncology 19(1):21–28. doi: 10.1002/pon.1556

Broderick JE, Junghaenel DU, Schneider S, Bruckenthal P, Keefe FJ (2011) Treatment expectation for pain coping skills training: relationship to osteoarthritis patients' baseline psychosocial characteristics (Clinical trial multicenter study randomized controlled trial research support, NIH, research support, non-US gov't). Clin J Pain 27(4):315–322. doi: 10.1097/AJP.0b013e3182048549

Brown CA, Seymour B, Boyle Y, El-Deredy W, Jones AK (2008) Modulation of pain ratings by expectation and uncertainty: behavioral characteristics and anticipatory neural correlates (Research support, non-US gov't). Pain 135(3):240–250. doi: 10.1016/j.pain.2007.05.022

Bultz BD, Carlson LE (2005) Emotional distress: the sixth vital sign in cancer care (Comp Stud Lett). J Clin Oncol 23(26):6440–6441. doi: 10.1200/JCO.2005.02.3259

Butt Z, Wagner LI, Beaumont JL, Paice JA, Peterman AH, Shevrin D, Cella D (2008) Use of a single-item screening tool to detect clinically significant fatigue, pain, distress, and anorexia in ambulatory cancer practice. J Pain Symptom Manage 35(1):20–30. doi: 10.1016/j.jpainsymman.2007.02.040

Calman KC (1984) Quality of life in cancer patients: an hypothesis. J Med Ethics 10(3):124–127

Chochinov HM, Hassard T, McClement S, Hack T, Kristjanson LJ, Harlos M, Murray A (2008) The patient dignity inventory: a novel way of measuring dignity-related distress in palliative care (Research support, non-US gov't). J Pain Symptom Manage 36(6):559–571. doi: 10.1016/j.jpainsymman.2007.12.018

Chochinov HM, Kristjanson LJ, Breitbart W, McClement S, Hack TF, Hassard T, Harlos, M (2011) Effect of dignity therapy on distress and end-of-life experience in terminally ill patients: a randomised controlled trial (Comparative study randomized controlled trial research support, NIH, extramural research support, non-US gov't). Lancet Oncol 12(8):753–762. doi: 10.1016/S1470-2045(11)70153-X

Cohen SR, Mount BM (2000) Living with cancer: "good" days and "bad" days: what produces them? Can the McGill quality of life questionnaire distinguish between them? (Research support, non-US gov't). Cancer 89(8):1854–1865

Cohen SR, Mount BM, Bruera E, Provost M, Rowe J, Tong K (1997) Validity of the McGill quality of life questionnaire in the palliative care setting: a multi-centre Canadian study demonstrating the importance of the existential domain (Research support, non-US gov't). Palliat Med 11(1):3–20

Colleoni M, Mandala M, Peruzzotti G, Robertson C, Bredart A, Goldhirsch A (2000) Depression and degree of acceptance of adjuvant cytotoxic drugs (Letter). Lancet 356(9238):1326–1327. doi:10.1016/S0140-6736(00)02821-X

Detering KM, Hancock AD, Reade MC, Silvester W (2010) The impact of advance care planning on end of life care in elderly patients: randomised controlled trial (Randomized controlled trial research support, non-US gov't). BMJ 340:c1345. doi: 10.1136/bmj.c1345

Eychmuller S (2012) SENS is making sense: on the way to an innovative approach to structure palliative care problems. Ther Umsch 69(2):87–90. doi:10.1024/0040-5930/a000256

Faller H, Bulzebruck H, Drings P, Lang H (1999) Coping, distress, and survival among patients with lung cancer (Research support, non-US gov't). Arch Gen Psychiatry 56(8):756–762

Fegg MJ, Kramer M, L'Hoste S, Borasio GD (2008) The schedule for meaning in life evaluation (SMiLE): validation of a new instrument for meaning-in-life research (Research support, non-US gov't validation studies). J Pain Symptom Manage 35(4):356–364. doi: 10.1016/j.jpainsymman.2007.05.007

Fox E (1997) Predominance of the curative model of medical care: a residual problem (Comment editorial). JAMA 278(9):761–763

Ganz PA (2008) Psychological and social aspects of breast cancer (Review). Oncology (Williston Park) 22(6):642–646, 650; discussion 650, 653

Herschbach P, Heusser P (2008) Einführung in die psychoonkologische Behandlungspraxis, 1st edn. Klett-Cotta, Stuttgart

Holland JC (2006) Psycho-oncology: from empirical research to screening program. In: Herschbach P, Heussner P, Sellschopp A (eds) *Psycho-onkologie, perspektiven heute* (pp 9–43): Pabst Science publishers

Holland JC, Andersen B, Breitbart WS, Dabrowski M, Dudley MM, Fleishman S, Zevon MA (2007) Distress management (Practice guideline). J Natl Compr Cancer Netw 5(1): 66–98

Junger S, Payne S (2011) Guidance on postgraduate education for psychologists involved in palliative care. Europ J Pall Care 18(5):238–252

Kissane DW, Clarke DM, Street AF (2001) Demoralization syndrome: a relevant psychiatric diagnosis for palliative care (Research support, non-US gov't review). J Palliat Care 17(1): 12–21

Kolva E, Rosenfeld B, Pessin H, Breitbart W, Brescia R (2011) Anxiety in terminally ill cancer patients (Research support, NIH, extramural). J Pain Symptom Manage 42(5):691–701. doi: 10.1016/j.jpainsymman.2011.01.013

Mitchell AJ, Chan M, Bhatti H, Halton M, Grassi L, Johansen C, Meader N (2011) Prevalence of depression, anxiety, and adjustment disorder in oncological, haematological, and palliative-care settings: a meta-analysis of 94 interview-based studies (Meta-analysis). Lancet Oncol 12(2):160–174. doi:10.1016/S1470-2045(11)70002-X

Mount B, Kearney M (2003) Healing and palliative care: charting our way forward (Editorial). Palliat Med 17(8):657–658

Nakazawa Y, Miyashita M, Morita T, Umeda M, Oyagi Y, Ogasawara T (2010) The palliative care self-reported practices scale and the palliative care difficulties scale: reliability and validity of two scales evaluating self-reported practices and difficulties experienced in palliative care by health professionals (Validation studies). J Palliat Med 13(4):427–437. doi: 10.1089/jpm.2009.0289

National Comprehensive Cancer Network (2003) Distress management clinical practice guidelines. J Natl Comp Cancer Network 1:344–374

Network NNCC (2003) Distress management: clinical practice guidelines (Practice guideline). J Natl Compr Cancer Netw 1(3):344–374

NICE (2011) The diagnosis and treatment of lung cancer (Update), vol 212. Cardiff (UK)

Nissim R, Gagliese L, Rodin G (2009) The desire for hastened death in individuals with advanced cancer: a longitudinal qualitative study (Research support, non-US gov't). Soc Sci Med 69(2):165–171. doi:10.1016/j.socscimed.2009.04.021

Parker PA, Baile WF, de Moor C, Cohen L (2003) Psychosocial and demographic predictors of quality of life in a large sample of cancer patients (Comparative study). Psychooncology 12(2):183–193. doi:10.1002/pon.635

Shipley V, Fairweather J (2001) A programme of individualized and self-administration of medicines in a hospice. Int J Palliat Nurs 7(12):581–586

Smith TJ, Temin S, Alesi ER, Abernethy AP, Balboni TA, Basch EM, Von Roenn JH (2012) American Society of Clinical Oncology provisional clinical opinion: the integration of palliative care into standard oncology care. J Clin Oncol 30(8):880–887. doi: 10.1200/JCO.2011.38.5161

Surbone A, Baider L, Weitzman TS, Brames MJ, Rittenberg CN, Johnson J (2010) Psychosocial care for patients and their families is integral to supportive care in cancer: MASCC position statement (Practice guideline). Support Care Cancer 18(2):255–263. doi:10.1007/s00520-009-0693-4

Temel JS, Greer JA, Admane S, Gallagher ER, Jackson VA, Lynch TJ, Pirl WF (2011) Longitudinal perceptions of prognosis and goals of therapy in patients with metastatic non-small-cell lung cancer: results of a randomized study of early palliative care (Randomized controlled trial research support, non-US gov't). J Clin Oncol 29(17):2319–2326. doi: 10.1200/JCO.2010.32.4459

Temel JS, Greer JA, Muzikansky A, Gallagher ER, Admane S, Jackson VA, Lynch TJ (2010) Early palliative care for patients with metastatic non-small-cell lung cancer (Randomized controlled trial research support, non-US gov't). N Engl J Med 363(8):733–742. doi: 10.1056/NEJMoa1000678

WHO (2002) Definition palliative care, 2013

Yoshida W, Seymour B, Koltzenburg M, Dolan RJ (2013) Uncertainty increases pain: evidence for a novel mechanism of pain modulation involving the periaqueductal gray. J Neurosci 33(13):5638–5646. doi:10.1523/JNEUROSCI.4984-12.2013

Zhang B, Wright AA, Huskamp HA, Nilsson ME, Maciejewski ML, Earle CC, Prigerson HG (2009) Health care costs in the last week of life: associations with end-of-life conversations (Research support, NIH, extramural research support, non-US gov't). Arch Intern Med 169(5):480-488. doi: 10.1001/archinternmed.2008.587

Psychosocial Burden of Family Caregivers to Adults with Cancer

Anna-leila Williams

Abstract

A person living with cancer will potentially have some degree of physical, cognitive, and/or psychological impairment, periods of unemployment, financial concerns, social isolation, and existential questions, any or all of which can impact the family and friends who surround them. In our current era of healthcare, patients with cancer receive invasive diagnostic studies and aggressive treatment as outpatients, and then convalesce at home. As such, cancer family caregivers are essential partners with the healthcare team. The intricacies of the cancer family caregiver role and responsibilities are demanding and may lead to increased morbidity and mortality—in effect, the cancer family caregiver can become a second patient in need of care. This chapter discusses the psychosocial burden of family caregivers to adults with cancer, and includes information on caregiver mood disturbance and psychological impairment and some of the mutable factors that contribute to these states (i.e., sleep disturbance, decline in physical health, and restriction of activities), uncertainty, spiritual concerns, and caregiver witnessing. There is a discussion of the factors that influence the caregiving experience (caregiver characteristics, patient characteristics, and social supports). The chapter concludes with comments on the state of caregiver research.

A. Williams (✉)
Frank H. Netter MD School of Medicine at Quinnipiac University, Hamden, Connecticut
e-mail: anna-leila.williams@quinnipiac.edu

Contents

1 Introduction.. 74
  1.1 Terminology... 74
  1.2 Why Focus on the Family Caregiver?.. 75
2 Mood Disturbance and Psychological Impairment 75
  2.1 Mutable Factors that Contribute to Mood Disturbance 78
3 Uncertainty.. 78
4 Spiritual Concerns 79
5 Caregiver Witnessing 79
6 Factors that Influence the Caregiving Experience................................... 81
  6.1 Caregiver Characteristics 80
  6.2 Patient Characteristics 81
  6.3 Caregiver Social Supports... 81
7 State of the Research... 81
8 Conclusion 82
References.. 82

1   Introduction

With almost 13 million people worldwide experiencing a cancer diagnosis in any given year (World Health Organization International Agency for Research on Cancer 2012), the consequences are far-reaching. A person living with cancer will potentially have some degree of physical, cognitive, and/or psychological impairment, periods of unemployment, financial concerns, social isolation, and existential questions, any or all of which can impact the family and friends who surround them.

1.1   Terminology

For the purpose of this discussion, the term *family caregiver* is defined as the primary person upon whom the patient relies for assistance with physical care, symptom management, and psychosocial needs, and who does not receive financial remuneration for caregiving (Seifert et al. 2008). This definition indicates the family caregiver does not need to be a blood or adoptive relative, nor a household member, and thus encompasses friends, neighbors, and relatives (such as adult children) who maintain separate homes.

The attention and subsequent volume of research devoted to cancer family caregivers has grown considerably over the past two decades. Unfortunately, a single definition of family caregiver has failed to emerge in the published literature. Several studies neglect to define the parameters for selection of their family caregiver study populations. Of those who provide a definition, a range of parameters have been expressed which encompass the caregiver's relationship to the patient, responsibilities, and/or household common with the patient. A subset of the cancer family caregiver definitions published in the research literature from 1993 to 2012 can be seen in Table 1. The consequences of not having a single definition for cancer family caregivers are many. Most notably, different study population sampling criteria likely contribute to inconsistent outcomes across studies. Obviously, the responsibilities (and consequent burdens) experienced by family caregivers who exclusively provide instrumental tasks, such as transportation and grocery shopping, are different than those experienced by family caregivers who address the patient's physical and psychological needs, such as wound care, bathing, medication management, and emotional support. As such, the ability to aggregate study outcomes, and have the cancer family caregiver research mature and progress has been stymied.

Throughout this chapter the author has deliberately avoided using the term "loved one" and instead uses the less emotionally charged terms "patient," "ill family member", and "person living with cancer." Caring for someone with cancer does not require love, nor does the process of caring necessarily engender love. Close interpersonal relations are enveloped in a spectrum of emotions, and the patient-caregiver dyad can be formed and the caregiver role undertaken for reasons other than love, including a sense of obligation, feelings of guilt, or financial concerns (Feinberg et al. 2006). To assume the cancer family caregiver and patient are "loved ones" denies the intensity of the dyad's relationship, and potentially constrains emotional expression from both parties.

1.2 Why Focus on the Family Caregiver?

Caring for someone who is ill is a ubiquitous behavior, common to our humanity throughout recorded time. So why do family caregivers deserve mention in a textbook of psycho-oncology if they are merely fulfilling a time honored human to human covenant? The answer is 2-fold. First, in our current era of healthcare, patients with cancer receive invasive diagnostic studies and aggressive treatment as outpatients, and then convalesce at home. As such, cancer family caregivers (who customarily receive little or no training from health professionals) are essential partners with the health care team, required to provide complex physical and psychological care, as well as help the patient navigate a complicated health care system and maintain the household (Blum and Sherman 2010). The intricacies of the cancer family caregiver role and responsibilities are demanding, therefore leading us to the second justification for focusing on family caregivers. We now have several decades' worth of descriptive data that identify the consequences of fulfilling the role of caregiver (Given et al. 2004; Harding and Higginson 2003; Park et al. 2010). The increased morbidity and mortality incurred by cancer family caregivers, some of which will be briefly described in this chapter, imply the family caregiver can be, in effect, a second patient in need of care (Northouse et al. 2012).

Table 1 A subset of cancer family caregiver definitions published in the research literature, 1993–2012

Study citation	Definitions
McCorkle et al. (1993)	"Biological family member or relative by marriage whom the patient identified as important."
Miaskowski et al. (1997)	"…identified by the patients as the individual most involved in their care."
Williamson et al. (1998)	"…(spouses who) have assumed meaningful responsibility for the day-to-day care of the patient without pay for the services they provided."
Grimm et al. (2000)	"…the nonprofessional person who helped the patient with physical care, symptom management, and coping…"
Cameron et al. (2002)	"…the person who conducted or coordinated the majority of the patient's home care needs without receiving financial reimbursement for the care they provided."
Northouse et al. (2002)	"…the family member or significant other identified by the patient as her primary source of emotional and physical support…"
Hwang et al. (2003)	"…a spouse, adult child, sibling, a parent of patient, or nonblood related person identified by the patient as the individual who is most involved in or affected by the patient's illness"
Matthews (2003)	"…unpaid, nonprofessional care providers who were members of the immediate family, distant relatives, or close friends."
Grunfeld et al. (2004)	"…a family member or friend who would be most responsible for on-going caregiving."
Gaugler et al. (2005)	"…provided help to a loved one because of cancer…"
Kim et al. (2006)	"…an individual in a family-like relationship who constantly provided help to (the person with cancer)."
Mellon et al. (2006)	"…family (member)/significant other over 18 years who had been through the cancer experience with (the patient) and had been (the patient's) main source of emotional or instrumental support."
Sherwood et al. (2006)	"…someone who provided ongoing support to the care recipient (including financial, emotional, and/or physical support)."
Walsh et al. (2007)	"…the main person who provided unpaid practical and emotional support to the patient on a regular basis and was in contact with the palliative care team."
Seifert et al. (2008)	"…someone who is involved with and helps the patient with his or her care and/or household activities; the caregiver was not necessarily a relative nor did he or she need to be living with the patient."
Hendrix et al. (2009)	"…an individual who lived in the same household as the cancer patient and provided the most "hands-on" care."

(continued)

Table 1 (continued)

Study citation	Definitions
O'Hara et al. (2010)	"… someone close to them (the patient) who was involved with their care…"
Beesley et al. (2011)	"The definition of caregiver was deliberately left for the patient to interpret however, when clarity was sought, a caregiver was described as someone who provided the patient with physical or emotional support. Paid caregivers were excluded."
Guay et al. (2012)	"…the spouse, first-degree relative, or other designated person who provides direct assistance to the patient in his or her activities of daily living."

2 Mood Disturbance and Psychological Impairment

Mood disturbances and psychological impairments are the most commonly explored variables in the cancer family caregiver literature. Researchers have used a variety of instruments to measure conceptual and diagnostic categorizations of psychological impairment, namely: anxiety, depression, stress, tension, strain, emotional well-being, and psychological distress (Williams and McCorkle 2011). The lack of a common metric makes it difficult to precisely assess the extent of psychological impairment among cancer family caregivers, and the subgroup of caregivers who are at greatest risk; however, it is noteworthy that, across almost all metrics, caregivers consistently have anxiety, depression, and psychological distress rates two or more times that of the general population (Kurtz et al. 2004; Grov et al. 2005; Grunfeld et al. 2004; Northouse et al. 2001; Williams et al. 2013). The lack of precision in the research literature around caregiver psychological impairment in no way obscures what is undoubtedly a major burden for cancer family caregivers. Several studies which concurrently measured psychological impairment in patients and family caregivers, found the family caregivers had higher rates of impairment than the patients with cancer (Braun et al. 2007; Kim et al. 2005; Matthews 2003; Mellon et al. 2006).

Cancer family caregiver mood disturbance and psychological impairment not only contribute to the caregiver's personal suffering, but also impact their relationship with the family member with cancer, and the care they are able to provide that family member. A wealth of data, compiled in two meta-analyses (Hagedoorn et al. 2000; Hodges et al. 2005) show mutual, bidirectional influences on psychological distress among the patient-caregiver dyad. A recent prospective, longitudinal study of patients with stage III or IV lung, gastrointestinal, or gynecological cancers and their family caregivers looked at the relationships among spirituality, health-related quality of life, and physical and psychological functioning. As expected, caregiver depression was inversely related to patient physical quality of life. Of interest, patient spiritual well-being mediated the relationship between patient physical quality of life and caregiver depression (Douglas and Daly 2012).

2.1   Mutable Factors that Contribute to Mood Disturbance

2.1.1   Sleep Disturbance

Several mutable factors contribute to cancer family caregivers' risk for mood disturbance. Similar to the general population, the cancer family caregiver population has an increased prevalence of anxiety and depression among those with disturbed sleep (Carter 2003; Carter and Acton 2006; Carter and Chang 2000; Gibbins et al. 2009). Cancer family caregivers, especially those who share a household with the ill family member, provide care 24 hours per day. Night time duties may include medication administration, toileting assistance, symptom management and support for treatment side-effects, as well as providing emotional support to the patient. As one would expect, disturbed sleep is a common concern for cancer family caregivers, with prevalence rates over 40 % (Gibbins et al. 2009).

2.1.2   Decline in Physical Health

Decline in the cancer family caregiver's physical health has been shown to contribute to an increased risk of depression among cancer family caregivers. A longitudinal study demonstrated decline in cancer family caregiver physical health over time is driven largely by the caregiver's perception of the caregiving experience (including their sense of social functioning and abandonment) and is a key determinant of depression (Kurtz et al. 2004). Cancer family caregiver physical health decline has been attributed to many factors including the stress and exhaustion of caring, and neglect of self-care and health maintenance because of prioritizing the patient (Carter 2003; Travis et al. 2004).

2.1.3   Restriction of Activities

Not surprisingly, as the cancer family caregiver's life becomes curtailed by caregiver responsibilities, there is an increased risk for mood disturbance and psychological impairment (Cameron et al. 2002; Williamson et al. 1998). When pleasurable and meaningful activities related to either work or leisure are usurped by the daily tasks and stressors of caring for someone with cancer, the cancer family caregiver's identity, coping strategies, self-care efforts, and social network may be disrupted (Cameron et al. 2002; Goldstein et al. 2004). The loss of pleasurable and meaningful activities can also add to the cancer family caregiver's perceived burden from caring (Kim et al. 2005), all of which increase the risk for mood disturbance and psychological impairment.

3   Uncertainty

Uncertainty is a constant companion for patients and family caregivers living with cancer throughout all stages of disease. Diagnosis, staging, treatment decisions, treatment related side-effects, disease and treatment monitoring, survivorship, recurrence, end of life—are all wrought with uncertainty and inflict turmoil on everyday life (Stajduhar et al. 2008; Temel et al. 2008). Patients and cancer family caregivers who are uncertain as to how the patient will feel or function in the near or distant future, have difficulty planning appointments, meals, work assignments, childcare responsibilities, social engagements, or vacations (Williams and Bakitas 2012). Essentially any activity or responsibility that takes planning requires a contingency because of the uncertainty of the patient's well-being. Managing uncertainty is a formidable trial for many people and cancer family caregivers are no exception. A 2009 qualitative study queried 33 bereaved and current cancer family caregivers of critically ill patients about what they felt was important for them to prepare for death and bereavement. Several factors related to life experience and cognitive, affective, and behavioral dimensions emerged as important to the caregivers. Notably, the participants *unanimously* reported uncertainty (as it relates to medical, psychosocial, religious/spiritual, and pragmatic issues) as their principal challenge; and identified communication as the chief means of managing uncertainty (Hebert et al. 2009).

4   Spiritual Concerns

The crucible of cancer family caregiving is laden with uncertainty, identity disruption, and physical and emotional challenges, and therefore, potentially provides the ideal environment for spiritual and existential questions to arise (Murray et al. 2010; Williams and Bakitas 2012). The literature on cancer family caregiver spirituality is small but burgeoning, and indicates spirituality may have been a potently influential variable that was overlooked in earlier research.

In a large national study, the American Cancer Society's Study of Cancer Survivors and Quality of Life Survey for Caregivers assessed spiritual wellbeing (defined as the ability to find meaning and peace) and its association with several patient and caregiver variables (Kim et al. 2011). Results show a significant association between spiritual wellbeing and mental health, for both patients and caregivers. Interestingly, when the caregivers in this study reported higher spiritual wellbeing, their family members with cancer reported better physical health. Determining whether patient physical health contributes to caregiver spirituality or vice versa, or if the relationship is bidirectional, awaits replication in longitudinal studies.

A recent small epidemiologic study of family caregivers to adults with advanced cancer enrolled in palliative care found *all* of the participants self-identified as "spiritual" and said their spirituality was a major means by which they coped with their family member's illness (Guay et al. 2012). That said, more than half of the participants reported they had "spiritual pain" [defined as 'a pain deep in your soul (being) that is not physical' (Mako et al. 2006)]. Participants who identified as having spiritual pain were significantly more likely to have elevated levels of anxiety, depression, denial, behavioral disengagement, and dysfunctional coping strategies than participants who did not identify spiritual pain. Of note, only 21 % of participants reported receiving supportive pastoral care services.

5   Caregiver Witnessing

Inherent in the family caregiver role is bearing witness to the plight of the person with cancer (Weitzner et al. 1999). The cancer family caregiver's journey with their ill family member begins with the shock of diagnosis and travels through the exploration of treatment decisions, the stress of managing symptoms and treatment side-effects, to the uncertainty of survivorship or the challenge of end of life and death. Beyond their personal experiences at each of the phases of disease, the cancer family caregiver often has the added task of witnessing the ill family member's ordeal of enduring aggressive care and its aftermath. The cancer family caregiver may have an intimate view of the patient's physical pain and deterioration, emotional anguish, and delerium. The consequences of witnessing for the family caregiver have not yet been fully explicated. Qualitative studies speak to the brutal reality of what cancer family caregivers witness (Murray et al. 2010; Stetz and Brown 1997; Williams and Bakitas 2012). A few epidemiologic studies have linked cancer family caregiver witnessing to their development of post-traumatic stress disorder and major depressive disorder (Barry et al. 2002; Wright et al. 2010).

The Yale Bereavement Study was the first study to evaluate the bereaved caregiver's perceptions of the patient's suffering during the illness, the violent nature of the death, and their sense of being prepared for the death, and how these factors are associated with major depressive disorder, post-traumatic stress disorder, and prolonged grief disorder (Barry et al. 2002). Earlier research classified deaths as violent based on how the death occurred (i.e., motor vehicle crash, homicide, suicide). The Yale Bereavement Study allowed the bereaved caregiver to classify the death as violent or peaceful, according to how much they perceived the patient to have pain and other physical symptoms. The authors, reporting on 122 bereaved adults who were interviewed at 4 months post-death (baseline) and 9 months post-death (follow-up), found perception of the death as violent led to a 1.5 times increased likelihood of major depressive disorder at baseline. A major limitation of The Yale Bereavement Study is its reliance on retrospective ratings of the bereaved person's perceptions, and the simultaneous evaluation of those ratings and assessment of the psychiatric diagnoses. It is possible individuals with post-death major depressive disorder and prolonged grief disorder may be inclined to perceive the circumstances surrounding the death negatively. Similarly, the directionality of the associations between the bereaved caregiver's perceptions and the psychiatric diagnoses is ambiguous. That said, The Yale Bereavement Study was a groundbreaking, ambitious and creative undertaking that laid the foundation for future research related to caregiver witnessing.

6 Factors that Influence the Caregiving Experience

6.1 Caregiver Characteristics

Much of the cancer family caregiver descriptive research has attempted to discern which factors influence the caregiving experience, either increasing or mitigating one's risk for psychosocial burden. While the assertion is often made that younger caregivers and female caregivers are at increased risk for developing anxiety and depression (Cameron et al. 2002; Given and Sherwood 2006; Kim and Given 2008; Pinquart and Sorensen 2003), there is also a body of literature that refutes these findings (Fenix et al. 2006; Gaston-Johnson et al. 2004; Goldstein et al. 2004; Grov et al. 2005; Williams et al. 2013). In all likelihood, the outcomes depend upon which variables the researchers chose to control for, such as socioeconomics, education, having other dependents in the household, employment status, and length of time as caregiver. Other minimally researched factors that might influence the caregiving experience include spirituality, religiosity, and personality trait (Fenix et al. 2006; Kim et al. 2005).

6.2 Patient Characteristics

Patient characteristics have been found to profoundly influence the cancer family caregiving experience. Caregivers caring for patients with greater physical decline, less functional ability, higher number of symptoms, and those who are close to death are at increased risk for psychological distress (Kim and Given 2008; Gaugler et al. 2005; Williams and McCorkle 2011). Also, if prior to the cancer diagnosis the dyad had a contentious relationship and/or communication difficulties, the caregiving experience is at increased risk for being antagonistic and contributing to caregiver mood disturbance (Kim and Carver 2007; Williams and Bakitas 2012).

6.3 Caregiver Social Supports

There is mounting evidence that the caregiving experience can be a time for personal growth and transformation, an opportunity to prioritize interpersonal relationships, heal old relational wounds, and reflect on and engage in meaningful and purposeful work (Colgrove et al. 2007; Moore et al. 2011). One factor that contributes to these positive aspects of caregiving may be the caregiver's social support network. It appears that if the caregiver has a supportive network of family and friends who can provide companionship, emotional support, instrumental care (meals, housecleaning, errands), and respite care, the cancer family caregiver can have the space and time necessary to garner perspective on the arduous role of caregiving (Williams and Bakitas 2012).

7   State of the Research

There is a sizable descriptive psychosocial assessment of cancer family caregivers accrued over the past 20 years. Several major problems with the literature are evident, namely: failure to set sampling parameters based on caregiver and patient characteristics; focus on psychosocial issues of family caregivers in isolation, rather than assessing the interrelationship between psychosocial, physical, and spiritual/existential needs; inattention to the dynamic nature of the caregiving role over time; and inconsistent use of measurement tools.

Clearly there is a need to standardize definitions and outcome measures used in cancer family caregiver research. The use of multiple measurement tools presents a major barrier to any type of comparative or aggregate analysis across studies, which is an essential next step in a field where most studies are comprised of small samples.

8   Conclusion

Cancer family caregivers are in the odd position of being essential members of the health care team, and having their own considerable health care needs. By supporting the caregiver, we in turn support the patient who invariably receives higher quality, more conscientious care at home.

References

Barry LC, Kasl SV, Prigerson HG (2002) Psychiatric disorders among bereaved persons: the role of perceived circumstances of death and preparedness for death. Am J Geriatr Psychiatry 10:447–457

Beesley VL, Price MA, Webb PM (2011) Loss of lifestyle: health behaviour and weight changes after becoming a caregiver of a family member diagnosed with ovarian cancer. Support Care Cancer 19:1949–1956

Blum K, Sherman DW (2010) Understanding the experience of caregivers: a focus on transition. Semin Ocol Nurs 26:243–258

Braun M, Mikulincer M, Rydall A, Walsh A, Rodin G (2007) Hidden morbidity in cancer: spouse caregivers. J Clin Oncol 25:4829–4834

Cameron J, Franche R, Cheung A, Stewart D (2002) Lifestyle interference and emotional distress in family caregivers of advanced cancer patients. Cancer 94:521–527

Carter P (2003) Family caregivers' sleep loss and depression over time. Cancer Nurs 26:253–259

Carter P, Chang B (2000) Sleep and depression in cancer caregivers. Cancer Nurs 23:410–415

Carter P, Acton GJ (2006) Personality and coping: predictors of depression and sleep problems among caregivers of individuals who have cancer. J Gerontol Nurs 32:45–53

Colgrove LA, Kim Y, Thompson N (2007) The effect of spirituality and gender on the quality of life of spousal caregivers of cancer survivors. Ann Behav Med 33:90–98

Douglas S, Daly BJ (2012) The impact of patient quality of life and spirituality upon caregiver depression for those with advanced cancer. Palliat Support Care. doi:10.1017/S14789515 12000570

Feinberg LF, Wolkwitz K, Goldstein C (2006) Ahead of the curve: emerging trends and practices in family caregiver support. AARP Public Policy Institute. http://assets.aarp.org/rgcenter/il/2006_09_caregiver.pdf. Accessed 20 April 2013

Fenix JB, Cherlin EJ, Prigerson HG, Johnson-Hurzeler R, Kasl SV, Bradley EH (2006) Religiousness and major depression among bereaved family caregivers: a 13-month follow-up study. J Palliat Care 22:286–292

Gaston-Johansson F, Lachica EM, Fall-Dickson JM, Kennedy MJ (2004) Psychological distress, fatigue, burden of care, and quality of life in primary caregivers of patients with breast cancer undergoing autologous bone marrow transplantation. Oncol Nurs Forum 31:1161–1169

Gaugler JE, Hanna N, Linder J, Given CW, Tolbert V, Kataria R, Regine WF (2005) Cancer caregiving and subjective stress: a multi-site, multi-dimensional analysis. Psychooncology 14:771–785

Gibbins J, McCoubrie R, Kendrick AH, Senior-Smith G, Davies AN, Hanks GW (2009) Sleep-wake disturbances in patients with advanced cancer and their family carers. J Pain Symptom Manage 38:860–870

Given B, Sherwood PR (2006) Family care for the older person with cancer. Semin Oncol Nurs 22:43–50

Given B, Wyatt G, Given C, Sherwood P, Gift A, DeVoss D, Rahbar M (2004) Burden and depression among caregivers of patients with cancer at the end of life. Oncol Nurs Forum 31:1105–1117

Goldstein M, Concato J, Fried T, Kasl S, Johnson-Hurzeler R, Bradley E (2004) Factors associated with caregiver burden among caregivers of terminally ill patients with cancer. J Palliat Care 20:38–43

Grimm PM, Zawacki KL, Mock V, Krumm S, Frink BB (2000) Caregiver responses and needs: an ambulatory bone marrow transplantation. Cancer Pract 8:120–128

Grov E, Dahl A, Moum T, Fossa S (2005) Anxiety, depression, and quality of life in caregivers of patients with cancer in late palliative phase. Annals Oncol 16:1185–1191

Grunfeld E, Coyle D, Whelan T, Clinch J, Reyno L, Earle C, Willan A, Viola R, Coristine M, Janz T, Glossop R (2004) Family caregiver burden: results of a longitudinal study of breast cancer patients and their principal caregivers. CMAJ 170:1795–1801

Guay M, Parsons HA, Hui D, De la Cruz MG, Thorney S, Bruera E (2012) Spirituality, religiosity, and spiritual pain among caregivers of patients with advanced cancer. Am J Hosp Palliat Care. doi:10.1177/1049909112458030

Hagedoorn M, Buunk BP, Kuijer RG, Wobbes T, Sanderman R (2000) Couples dealing with cancer: role and gender differences regarding psychological distress and quality of life. Psychooncology 9:232–242

Harding R, Higginson I (2003) What is the best way to help caregivers in cancer and palliative care? a systematic literature review of interventions and their effectiveness. Palliat Med 17:63–74

Hebert RS, Schulz R, Copeland VC, Arnold RM (2009) Preparing family caregivers for death and bereavement: insights from caregivers of terminally ill patients. J Pain Symptom Manage 37:3–12

Hendrix CC, Abernethy A, Sloane R, Misuraca J, Moore J (2009) A pilot study on the influence of an individualized and experiential training on cancer caregiver's self-efficacy in home care and symptom management. Home Health Nurse 27:271–278

Hodges J, Humphries G, MacFarlane G (2005) A meta-analytic investigation of the relationship between the psychological distress of cancer patients and their carers. Soc Sci Med 60:1–12

Hwang SS, Chang VT, Alejandro Y, Osenenko P, Davis C, Cogswell J, Srinivas S, Kasimis B (2003) Caregiver unmet needs, burden, and satisfaction in symptomatic advanced cancer patients at a veterans affairs medical center. Palliat Support Care 1:319–329

Kim Y, Baker F, Spillers RL, Wellisch DK (2006) Psychological adjustment of cancer caregivers with multiple roles. Psychooncology 15:795–804

Kim Y, Carver CS (2007) Frequency and difficulty in caregiving among spouses of individuals with cancer: effects of adult attachment and gender. Psychooncology 12:714–723

Kim Y, Carver CS, Spillers RL, Crammer C, Zhou ES (2011) Individual and dyadic relations between spiritual well-being and quality of life among cancer survivors and their spousal caregivers. Psychooncology 20:762–770

Kim Y, Duberstin PR, Sorensen S (2005) Levels of depressive symptoms in spouses of people with lung cancer: effects of personality, social support, and caregiving burden. Psychosomatics 46:123–130

Kim Y, Given BA (2008) Quality of life of family caregivers of cancer survivors: across the trajectory of the illness. Cancer 112(11 Suppl):2556–2568

Kurtz M, Kurtz J, Given C, Given B (2004) Depression and physical health among family caregivers of geriatric patients with cancer—a longitudinal view. Med Sci Monit 10:CR447–456

Mako C, Gale K, Poppito SR (2006) Spiritual pain among patients with advanced cancer in palliative care. J Palliat Med 9:1106–1113

Matthews BA (2003) Role and gender differences in cancer-related distress: a comparison of survivor and caregiver self-reports. Oncol Nurs Forum 30:493–499

McCorkle R, Yost LS, Jepson C, Malone D, Baird S, Lusk E (1993) A cancer experience: relationship of patient psychosocial responses to care-giver burden over time. Psychooncology 2:21–32

Mellon S, Northouse LL, Weiss LK (2006) A population-based study of the quality of life of cancer survivors and their family caregivers. Cancer Nurs 29:120–131

Miaskowski C, Kragness L, Dibble S, Wallhagen M (1997) Differences in mood states, health status, and caregiver strain between family caregivers of oncology outpatients with and without cancer-related pain. J Pain Symptom Manage 13:138–147

Moore AM, Gamblin TC, Geller DA, Youssef MN, Hoffman KE, Gemmell L, Likumahuwa SM, Bovbjerg DH, Marsland A, Steel JL (2011) A prospective study of posttraumatic growth as assessed by self-report and family caregiver in the context of advanced cancer. Psychooncology 20:479–487

Murray SA, Kendall M, Boyd K, Grant L, Highet G, Sheikh A (2010) Archetypal trajectories of social, psychological, and spiritual well-being and distress in family care givers of patients with lung cancer. BMJ 304:c2581

Northouse L, Mood D, Kershaw T, Schafenacker A, Mellon S, Walker J, Galvin E, Decker V (2002) Quality of life of women with recurrent breast cancer and their family members. J Clin Oncol 20:4050–4064

Northouse L, Templin T, Mood D (2001) Couples' adjustment to breast disease during the first year following diagnosis. J Behave Med 24:115–136

Northouse L, Williams AL, Given B, McCorkle R (2012) Psychosocial care for family caregivers of patients with cancer. J Clin Oncol 30:1227–1234

O'Hara RE, Hull JG, Lyons KD, Bakitas M, Hegel MT, Li Z, Ahles TA (2010) Impact on caregiver burden of a patient-focused palliative care intervention for patients with advanced cancer. Palliat Support Care 8:395–404

Park SM, Kim YJ, Kim S, Choi JS, Lim HY, Choi YS, Hong YS, Kim SY, Heo DS, Kang KM, Jeong HS, Lee CG, Moon DH, Choi JY, Kong IS, Yun YH (2010) Impact of caregivers' unmet needs for supportive care on quality of terminal cancer care delivered and caregiver's workforce performance. Support Care Cancer 18:699–706

Pinquart M, Sorensen S (2003) Differences between caregivers and noncaregivers in psychological health and physical health: a meta-analysis. Psychol Aging 18:250–267

Seifert ML, Williams AL, Dowd MF, Chappel-Aiken L, McCorkle R (2008) The caregiving experience in a racially diverse sample of cancer family caregivers. Cancer Nurs 31:399–407

Sherwood PR, Given BA, Given CW, Schiffman RF, Murman DL, Lovely M, von Eye A, Rogers LR, Remcr S (2006) Predictors of distress in caregivers of persons with a primary malignant brain tumor. Res Nurs Health 29:105–120

Stajduhar KI, Martin WL, Barwich D, Fyles G (2008) Factors influencing family caregivers' ability to cope with providing end-of-life cancer care at home. Cancer Nurs 31:77–85

Stetz KM, Brown MA (1997) Taking care: caregiving to persons with cancer and AIDS. Cancer Nurs 20:12–22

Temel JS, McCannon J, Greer JA, Jackson, VA, Ostler P, Pirl WF, Lynch TJ, Billings JA (2008) Aggressiveness of care in a prospective cohort of patients with advanced NSCLC. Cancer 113:826–833

Travis LA, Lyness JM, Shields CG, King DA, Cox C (2004) Social support, depression, and functional disability in older adult primary-care patients. Am J Geriatr Psychiatry 12:265–271

Walsh K, Jones L, Tookman A, Mason C, McLoughlin J, Blizard R (2007) Reducing emotional distress in people caring for patients receiving specialist palliative care. Br J Psychiatr 190:142–147

Weitzner MA, McMillan SC, Jacobsen PB (1999) Family caregiver quality of life: differences between curative and palliative cancer treatment settings. J Pain Symptom Manage 17:418–428

Williams AL, Bakitas M (2012) Cancer family caregivers: a new direction for interventions. J Palliat Med 15:775–783

Williams AL, Holmes-Tisch AJ, Dixon J, McCorkle R (2013) Factors associated with depressive symptoms in cancer family caregivers of patients receiving chemotherapy. Support Care Cancer. doi:10.1007/s00520-013-1802-y

Williams AL, McCorkle R (2011) Cancer family caregivers during the palliative, hospice, and bereavement phases: a review of the descriptive psychosocial literature. Palliat Support Care 9:315–325

Williamson G, Shaffer D, Schulz R (1998) Activity restriction and prior relationship history as contributors to mental health outcomes among middle-aged and older spousal caregivers. Health Psychol 17:152–162

World Health Organization International Agency for Research on Cancer (2012) World cancer factsheet. http://publications.cancerresearchuk.org/downloads/product/CS_FS_WORLD_A4.pdf. Accessed 13 April 2013

Wright AA, Keating NL, Balboni TA, Matulonis UA, Block SD, Prigerson HG (2010) Place of death: correlations with quality of life of patients with cancer and predictors of bereaved caregivers' mental health. J Clin Oncol 28:4457–4464

Rehabilitation for Cancer Patients

Joachim Weis and Jürgen M. Giesler

Abstract

Rehabilitation for cancer patients aims at reducing the impact of disabling and limiting conditions resulting from cancer and its treatment in order to enable patients to regain social integration and participation. Given current trends in cancer incidence and survival along with progress in medical treatment, cancer rehabilitation is becoming increasingly important in contemporary healthcare. Although not without limitations, the International Classification of Functioning, Disability, and Health (ICF) provides a valuable perspective for cancer rehabilitation in understanding impairments in functioning and activity as the result of an interaction between a health condition and contextual factors. The structure of cancer rehabilitation varies across countries as a function of their health care systems and social security legislations, although there is a broad consensus with respect to its principal goals. Cancer rehabilitation requires a careful assessment of the individual patient's rehabilitation needs and a multidisciplinary team of health professionals. A variety of rehabilitation interventions exist, including psycho-oncological and psycho-educational approaches. Research on the effectiveness of cancer rehabilitation provides evidence of improvements in relevant outcome parameters, but faces some methodological challenges as well.

J. Weis (✉) · J. M. Giesler
Klinik für Tumorbiologie an der Albert-Ludwigs-Universität Freiburg,
Psychosoziale Abteilung, Tumor Biology Center at the University of Freiburg,
Psychosocial Department, Breisacher Str. 117, 79106, Freiburg, Germany
e-mail: weis@tumorbio.uni-freiburg.de

J. M. Giesler
e-mail: giesler@tumorbio.uni-freiburg.de

U. Goerling (ed.), *Psycho-Oncology*, Recent Results in Cancer Research 197,   87
DOI: 10.1007/978-3-642-40187-9_7, © Springer-Verlag Berlin Heidelberg 2014

Contents

1   Increasing Relevance of Rehabilitation in Cancer.. 88
2   Focus and Basic Concepts of Cancer Rehabilitation... 89
3   Structure of Rehabilitation Care 90
4   Rehabilitation Needs and Assessment 92
5   Goals and Interventions.. 93
6   Psycho-Oncology in Rehabilitation 94
7   Cancer Rehabilitation: A Multidisciplinary Task 95
8   Evaluation of Cancer Rehabilitation... 96
9   Summary and Outlook 98
References... 98

1   Increasing Relevance of Rehabilitation in Cancer

As has been well documented (Bray et al. 2012), cancer incidence continues to rise worldwide as does the number of cancer survivors. For the year 2008, e.g., the International Agency for Research on Cancer (IARC) estimates that about 12.7 million people have been diagnosed with cancer all over the world (Cancer Research UK 2011; Ferlay et al. 2010). For the same year, the 5-years-prevalence of cancer worldwide has been estimated with 29 million persons (Cancer Research UK 2012). By the year 2030, the number of persons newly diagnosed with cancer is annually expected to rise to about 22 million (Cancer Research UK 2012). Irrespective of considerable variation between different countries in these parameters, these trends reflect the effects of various factors. Among these, advances in medical treatment and early detection of cancer during the past three decades as well as the increasingly higher life expectancy of the population play a significant role. In addition, changes in life-style associated with the development of modern industrialized societies have to be taken into account here. As a consequence of these trends, an increasing number of persons will require medical treatment for cancer, long-term surveillance, and eventually palliative care in the future. Thus, cancer has turned into a life-threatening chronic condition for a large proportion of patients that poses new challenges for comprehensive cancer care. These include, among others, a change in patient role toward more active participation in treatment decisions and treatment itself depending on the individual patients' needs and expectations.

Oncologic treatment typically includes surgery, chemotherapy, and/or radiation which in general have become increasingly more complex, long lasting as well as more invasive. That is, treatment may produce significant toxicities which cause substantial short- and long-term side effects, functional loss in various behavioral and life domains (physical, cognitive, emotional, social, and vocational) as well as psychosocial distress. Quality of life and functional status for a considerable proportion of patients will thus be substantially reduced. Against this background, cancer rehabilitation may generally be defined as the coordinated efforts of health care professionals to help patients overcome, minimize, or compensate the functional impairments and activity limitations brought about by the disease and its treatment. Due to the different developments described above, the importance of cancer rehabilitation has steadily increased during the past decades. Thus, rehabilitation has become an increasingly essential part in comprehensive cancer care covering the entire continuum from early detection, diagnosis, primary and adjuvant treatment, survivorship, and aftercare to end-of-life phases.

2   Focus and Basic Concepts of Cancer Rehabilitation

If one follows the WHO's definition of rehabilitation in general (WHO 1981), cancer rehabilitation may be understood as the "use of all means at reducing the impact of disabling and handicapping conditions" associated with cancer and its treatment with the aim of enabling patients to regain physical, social, psychological, and work-related functionality and "to achieve optimal social integration" (see also Gerber 2001; Gerber et al. 2005, Meyer et al. 2011). This process starts already during or immediately after the end of the primary treatment in terms of secondary and tertiary prevention.

Basic to this understanding of cancer rehabilitation is a concept of functional health that the International Classification of Functioning, Disability, and Health (ICF) of the WHO (2001; German version: Deutsches Institut für Medizinische Dokumentation und Information 2005) builds upon. From this perspective, a person would be considered functionally healthy if his/her body functions are in accordance with accepted norms, if he/she can do what a person without a health condition would be expected to be able to do, and if he/she could live his/her life in personally important life domains in a way as it would be expected of a person without functional impairments and restrictions to activities and participation.

As can be seen from Fig. 1, the ICF distinguishes between health conditions and contextual factors. Thus, it provides a new perspective on disability and functional impairment which are now explicitly viewed as outcomes of an *interaction* between these health conditions and contextual factors. This perspective integrates a social and a biomedical model of disability into a biopsychosocial one. In addition, Fig. 1 shows that the ICF distinguishes between body functions and structures, activities and participation in order to describe levels of restricted functioning. *Body functions* refer to physiological functions of body systems (including psychological functions), whereas *body structures* comprise anatomical parts of the body such as organs, limbs, and their components. Problems at this level may take the form of significant deviation or loss and are termed *impairments*. On the next level, activity means the execution of a task or an action by an individual and difficulties in executing tasks are termed *activity limitations*. Finally, *participation* refers to a person's involvement in a life situation and problems experienced by the individual in this respect are referred to as *participation restrictions*. *Environmental factors* (comprising a person's physical, social

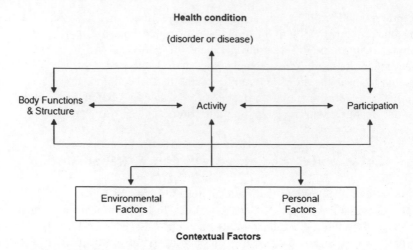

Fig. 1 Model of disability underlying the ICF (WHO 2001)

and attitudinal environment) and *personal factors* (e.g., a person's optimism) may moderate how a given health condition impacts on the three levels of functioning and activity and thus on the manifestation of disability. As an example in the field of cancer, one might consider the case of a patient with peripheral neuropathy and ankle weakness resulting from chemotherapy (Gilchrist et al. 2009). This might lead to a limitation in this patient's ability to walk. However, whether or not this would result in a participation restriction in the vocational domain as well would of cause depend on the person's vocation (e.g., if he were a fire fighter as opposed to a computer programmer).

Intended as a complement to the International Classification of Diseases (ICD), the ICF provides an extensive set of categories by which a person's functional impairments, activity restrictions, and limitations deriving from a health condition may be described in detail with additional reference to contextual factors. To be clinically useful, however, subsets of this extensive list have to be built which refer to specific health conditions and represent so-called ICF core sets. In the field of cancer, core sets for breast as well as for head and neck cancer have been developed and are currently undergoing validation (Becker et al. 2010; Brach et al. 2004; Glaessel et al. 2011; Leib et al. 2012; Tschiesner et al. 2009, 2010). This research lends support to the content validity of the respective core set categories on the one hand, but on the other also identifies the need for further amendments. Thus, there still is a need for additional development and further validation. Although the general perspective provided by ICF has been positively evaluated so far, it remains to be seen, then, whether core sets covering impairments and limitations associated with other tumor diagnoses will emerge. Furthermore, reservations concerning the applicability and practicability of ICF categories in the field of cancer rehabilitation (e.g., Bornbaum et al. 2013) will have to be resolved.

3   Structure of Rehabilitation Care

Considering the continuum of cancer care, cancer rehabilitation has its place at the interface of acute and follow-up or after-care. How rehabilitation services are delivered varies greatly from country to country as a function of the social security system into which they are embedded. In most European countries and in the United States of America rehabilitation services are mostly based in out-patient settings, whereas in Germany one finds a unique system in which rehabilitation services are provided predominantly through in-patient settings although out-patient rehabilitation services have partially gained importance there in recent years, too.

Hellbom et al. (2011) recently have provided a brief overview of the structures of cancer rehabilitation and the state of rehabilitation research in Nordic and European countries. As they point out, cancer rehabilitation ranges from primarily out-patient programs as in Sweden, Norway, and the Netherlands over 1-week courses as in Finland, Denmark, Iceland and, again, Sweden and Norway to (predominantly in-patient) 3-week programs in Germany (for Germany see also Koch and Morfeld 2004; Koch et al. 2000; Koch and Weis 1992).

One of many interesting characteristics of the German rehabilitation system is that rehabilitation costs are primarily covered by the German statutory pension insurance scheme or the patient's health insurance–depending on whether or not the patient still is in the labor force. Different from patients with other health conditions, however, cancer patients in Germany generally are entitled to apply for rehabilitation measures. Rehabilitation of cancer patients not yet retired is guided by the aim of restoring their earning capacity (as a prerequisite of social participation) which is well captured by the official slogan "rehabilitation rather then pension". Another specific feature of rehabilitation in Germany is a special form of rehabilitation that is termed "post-acute rehabilitation." This refers formally to rehabilitation services that are about to begin not later than 2 weeks after discharge from the acute-care hospital. This type of rehabilitation measures represented about 35 % of all rehabilitation measures in 2011 (Deutsche Rentenversicherung Bund 2012b).

In 2011, the German statutory pension insurance scheme provided a total of 163,466 in- and out-patient cancer rehabilitation measures (Deutsche Rentenversicherung Bund 2012b). These represent 18 % of all its rehabilitation measures for adults in that year. 84 % of all rehabilitation measures in 2011 were in-patient measures and 13 % were out-patient measures (both for adults). The latter represents an increase of 7 % points over 16 years. This mainly reflects the efforts that have been taken during that time in order to develop out-patient services in Germany, too, in order to tailor services more specifically to the needs of some subgroups of the patient population. However, with respect to the total of in-patient rehabilitation measures provided in 2011 in approximately 120 oncologic rehabilitation clinics the proportions of women and men amounted to 21 and 16 %, respectively, while the proportion of patients with cancer in regard to the total of out-patient rehabilitation measures amounted to only 2 % in both women and men.

In the United States of America, the form of delivering cancer rehabilitation has undergone some notable changes during the past decades according to observations by Alfano et al. (2012). These authors note a shift in rehabilitation service delivery away from tertiary cancer centers to community centers coupled with a fragmentation of cancer care in community settings. In combination, these trends limit the potential of cancer rehabilitation. In order to improve this unsatisfactory situation Alfano et al. (2012) suggest to revitalize the link between primary treatment and rehabilitation services and also to consider the possibility to integrate some elements of the European forms of rehabilitation into the US system of health care. It remains to be seen how this will translate into practice. Nevertheless, these recommendations fit well with initiatives of the Institute of Medicine to establish the concept of a cancer survivorship plan that describes the tasks for survivorship care of any individual patient (Oeffinger and McCabe 2006; Salz et al. 2012; Stout et al. 2012).

So far, this section should have made clear that the structure of delivering cancer rehabilitation not only varies widely across countries, but also is undergoing dynamic processes of change in response to changes in medical care and society in general. Despite the marked variation in the delivery of cancer rehabilitation services across different countries, however, there appears to be a general consensus that cancer rehabilitation is a multidisciplinary task (for details see Sect. 7).

4 Rehabilitation Needs and Assessment

Physical and psychosocial sequelae of cancer and its treatment differ widely between patients and the stages of the cancer trajectory. Problems during the initial phase immediately after treatment are different from those that may arise in later phases, e.g., after a recurrence or at the end of life (Gerber 2001). More specifically, the spectrum of sequelae may include fear of recurrence, anxiety, depression, cognitive dysfunction, fatigue, pain syndromes, peripheral neuropathy, sexual dysfunction, problems with body image, balance and gait problems, various mobility issues, lymphedema, problems with bladder and bowel functioning, stoma care, problems with swallowing, and speech and communication difficulties (Alfano et al. 2012; Fialka-Moser et al. 2003; Stubblefield and O'Dell 2009). Given this broad range of potential impairments in combination with the wide variability between patients, each cancer patient requesting rehabilitation has to be assessed individually with respect to his/her rehabilitation needs (Gamble et al. 2011; Ruppert et al. 2010). This assessment will take place routinely at admission in terms of a medical examination and interview. It may be complemented by a short psychological assessment by a psychologist or on the basis of a routine distress screening procedure. Determining a patient's rehabilitation needs could be improved using standardized instruments designed to measure quality of life. These may be either generic or may focus on the specific problems and distress of cancer patients. Aside from assisting in the assessment of rehabilitation needs before or at admission, these instruments may be used efficiently in evaluating the effects of rehabilitation programs at discharge or follow-up examinations as well. Schag et al. (1991) and Ganz et al. (1992) were among the first to develop a comprehensive instrument for assessing rehabilitation needs in cancer patients. Overviews of more recent instruments may be obtained from a variety of sources (e.g., Mpofu and Oakland 2010). Bengel et al. (2008) have provided an update of instruments available to assessments in rehabilitation in Germany, covering internationally established ones for which a validated German version exists as well as instruments available only in German. Table 1 illustrates some of the more frequently used instruments that are generally available to assessments in cancer rehabilitation settings.

5 Goals and Interventions

Given the multifaceted impairments and sequelae due to cancer and its treatment, cancer rehabilitation usually addresses a variety of goals. On a general level, cancer rehabilitation aims at restoring the patient's physical, emotional, social, role, and cognitive functioning as well as independence. This may also include re-integration into work life. Besides helping the patient regain functional autonomy, preventing further impairment of functioning may frequently represent another important task for rehabilitation of cancer patients. Following a suggestion by Bergelt and Koch (2002) rehabilitation goals may be classified as biomedical/treatment-related, psychosocial, educational, or vocational. Table 2 presents an illustrative list of rehabilitation goals covering these categories.

Specifying rehabilitation goals for the individual patient will take his/her individual needs into account as well as the results of all other assessments. In addition, the goals to be specified should be attainable within a reasonable amount of time. Based on this principle and the respective assessments an individual rehabilitation plan will be developed in close cooperation with the patient. Also,

Table 1 Illustrative selection of instruments and domains available to assessment in cancer rehabilitation

Domain	Instruments
Quality of life	*Cancer specific:* EORTC QLQ-C30, FACIT, *Generic:* NHP, SF-36
Health-related cognitions	IPQ-R, MHLC, SOC
Coping with cancer	CBI, COPE, FKV*, TSK*, WoCL
Social support	ISSS, SSUK*
Pain	MPI, PDI
Distress/co-morbidity	BDI-II, BSI, DT, GHQ, HADS

Note *Available only in German

Table 2 Types of intervention goals in cancer rehabilitation (slightly modified after Bergelt and Koch 2002)

Biomedical/treatment-related goals
To continue therapies as recommended after primary treatment
To identify and treat sequelae of cancer and its treatment (e.g., pain, fatigue, lack of endurance, peripheral neuropathy, sleep disorders)
To improve physical condition and performance status focusing on strength, endurance, and mobility
Psychosocial goals
To support the process of coping with the disease and the accompanying physical changes
To restore and improve social, emotional, and cognitive functioning
To enhance self help strategies, competencies and resources for disease management
To facilitate adaptation to irreversible limitations and help the patient develop compensatory skills and abilities
To help the patient stabilize with respect to his/her personal, familial, social, and vocational situation
Educational goals
To provide information on cancer, its treatment, and forms of psychosocial support
To provide information on risk factors and to initiate modification in health-related behaviors like dietary habits, exercise, smoking, or alcohol consumption
Vocational goals
To help the patient achieve vocational re-integration, resume previous occupation, or retrain in order to attain a position appropriate under given circumstances

patients and–wherever possible and indicated–their family will be encouraged to actively participate as partners in the rehabilitation process and thus contribute to attain its goals. In the end, the rehabilitation plan will combine a variety of medical and psychosocial interventions considered necessary to achieve the specified objectives. As an illustration, Table 3 presents an overview of the treatment options typically available in cancer rehabilitation programs.

In addition, specialized programs have been developed that address issues and sequelae of patients from a given diagnostic or treatment subgroup (e.g., patients with breast or prostate cancer or patients having undergone stem cell transplantation). Thus, rehabilitation programs designed specifically for women with breast cancer may, e.g., focus on comprehensive management of lymphedema, exercise, dietary counseling, post-operative management of breast reconstruction, psychological counseling or psychotherapy, and dance therapy in order to address problems with body image and self-esteem. Similarly, patients suffering from severe fatigue and decreased physical performance for a prolonged period of recovery after having received stem cell transplantation may also profit from a specialized program that might combine elements of physical exercise and psycho-educational interventions.

Table 3 Interventions in cancer rehabilitation	Medical treatment including pain management and complementary medicine
	Physical therapy and exercise programs
	Diet counseling
	Smoking cessation education
	Psychological counseling/individual psychotherapy
	Psycho-education
	Art therapy/occupational therapy
	Neuropsychological training

6 Psycho-Oncology in Rehabilitation

Psycho-oncological interventions are well recognized as an essential part of a comprehensive cancer rehabilitation program. They address the cognitive, behavioral, and emotional facets of the patients' (and their families') response to cancer and its treatment. During the past decades numerous psycho-oncological interventions based on individual or group therapy approaches have been developed (Newell et al. 2002; Holland et al. 2010), which are carried out also in rehabilitation centers. As meta-analyses and systematic reviews have shown, evidence of the effectiveness of these interventions is available at the high ranking EBM levels I or II (NHMRC 2003; Faller et al. 2013; Edwards et al. 2008). In a rehabilitation setting, psycho-educational group interventions are utilized to address the patients' psychosocial distress and to give participants the opportunity to share their experiences and find a solution to their problems. These interventions are frequently based on a cognitive–behavioral approach and include various elements as summarized in Table 4. They typically encompass 4 to 12 sessions with a maximum of 10 to 12 patients each. These interventions are operated on the basis of a structured agenda that focuses on the most prevalent issues of cancer patients and aim at initiating an active coping behavior.

Table 4 Elements of psycho-educational programs in cancer rehabilitation	Information about cancer and its treatment
	Social and emotional support, sharing of experience
	Stress management
	Cognitive–behavioral self-instruction and self-control techniques
	Relaxation, guided imagery

7   Cancer Rehabilitation: A Multidisciplinary Task

Due to the multifaceted nature of cancer and its treatment, cancer rehabilitation requires a multidisciplinary team of health care professionals (Alfano et al. 2012; Hellbom et al. 2011; Ruppert et al. 2010). The interventions provided by these professionals in accordance with an individual patient's rehabilitation plan have to be coordinated by a member of the team who in most cases will be the rehabilitation physician. The multidisciplinary cancer rehabilitation team may thus include members from the following professions: oncology, psychology, nursing, nutritional counseling, physiotherapy and physical therapy, occupational therapy, art therapy (including music therapy, dance therapy, etc.), social work/vocational counseling as well as spiritual care. As a team, these professionals work together very closely, thus requiring a regularly based professional interchange in terms of multidisciplinary case conferences across the course of rehabilitation. In addition, external supervision will support the work of the multidisciplinary cancer rehabilitation team as a well established instrument of quality assurance.

8   Evaluation of Cancer Rehabilitation

Cost-effectiveness has become a major issue in healthcare and rehabilitation services over the past years. As a consequence, evaluating the effectiveness and efficiency of rehabilitation in general and cancer rehabilitation in particular has also become a major field of research over the past three decades wherever health care systems are providing rehabilitation services. Efforts at addressing the effectiveness of rehabilitation services empirically may also be useful in providing a basis for attempts at implementing programs for quality assurance in rehabilitation settings.

Evaluation of cancer rehabilitation may be carried out at the level of single intervention modules of which a rehabilitation program is made up and at the level of multicomponent programs as whole. Thus, evaluation of cancer rehabilitation covers the whole spectrum from randomized controlled studies of specific interventions to health-services research addressing the effects of established programs at more complex levels. However, while randomization may be easily performed when evaluating single interventions, randomization may be difficult to perform at the level of evaluation a program as a whole.

For the majority of the countries focused upon by Hellbom et al. (2011), studies on the effectiveness of rehabilitation interventions for cancer patients are available. However, these authors also support the assumption that the level of available evidence of the effectiveness of single interventions in rehabilitation settings varies–with largely positive results for interventions like relaxation training or psychosocial counseling, whereas evidence levels are lower for effects of interventions like, e.g., lymph drainage or art therapy (Weis and Domann 2006). Similarly, higher levels of evidence appear to be available for interventions targeting fatigue and physical exercise (Cramp and Byron-Daniel 2012; Mishra et al. 2012; Puetz et al. 2012; Spelten et al. 2003; Spence et al. 2007; van Weert et al. 2005, 2006, 2010). With respect to the rehabilitation of patients with prostate cancer, however, Hergert et al. (2009) report rather limited evidence of the effectiveness of the majority of the interventions investigated by the studies they reviewed. As a consequence, these authors suggest additional and methodologically stronger research in this field of rehabilitation.

In Germany, efforts at establishing quality assurance and research programs in rehabilitation settings started in the 1980s. As a result, various means of quality assurance have been implemented (expert visitations of rehabilitation centers, expert reviews of discharge records and recommendations, and patient surveys) and are considered to be working successfully. Regarding the effectiveness of cancer rehabilitation at the program level earlier as well as more recent research in Germany provides evidence of patients improving with respect to health-related quality of life, subjective well-being and physical functioning or symptoms (Bartsch et al. 2003; Heim et al. 2001; Krüger et al. 2009; Schwiersch et al. 1994; Teichmann 2002; Weis and Domann 2006). In general, rehabilitation effects found for patients with cancer or other chronic conditions in Germany have been interpreted as clinically meaningful (Haaf 2005). That rehabilitation measures are cost-effective as well may probably also be assumed insofar as it can be shown that the costs for rehabilitation reach the break-even point if a person's retirement may be postponed for at least 4 months (Deutsche Rentenversicherung Bund 2012a).

As a comparative study by Weis et al. (2006) showed, patients with non-metastatic breast cancer receiving rehabilitation differed from a group of comparable patients not planning to have rehabilitation by lower emotional functioning, higher psychosocial distress, and more disease-specific impairments. This was taken to indicate that processes of (adequate) referral by health-professionals and self-selection by patients themselves were in operation as might have been expected in light of the objectives of rehabilitation. In addition, controlling for the influence of prior chemotherapy, Weis et al. (2006) found improvements in their patients with respect to health-related quality of life, anxiety, and depression as measured by the HADS, and in specific symptoms. When compared to the patients not attending cancer rehabilitation, effects of the factor "treatment/time of assessment" were mainly found to be of moderate size and higher for patients having received rehabilitation.

Although the available evidence thus suggests positive effects of cancer rehabilitation, there still are some unresolved issues and challenges to be addressed by future research. One of these issues concerns the question whether the improvements reported for various outcome parameters during rehabilitation are sufficiently stable beyond discharge. In fact, some studies have reported a decrease of health-related quality of life or well-being after discharge and initial improvements—in some cases to even lower levels than those observed at admission (e.g., Weis et al. 2006). Consequently, further research is needed in order to clarify whether improvement or deterioration across time vary as a function of the demands of the rehabilitation program, the transfer of newly acquired skills to daily life, the disease, socio-demographic characteristics, and the patient's social and psychological status. Another issue, of course, is the fact that the majority of studies to date do not employ a randomized controlled design that alone would allow causal inferences. Therefore, setting up valid designs whenever randomized control is not feasible will continue to present a major challenge for researchers in the field of cancer rehabilitation who are interested in causal inferences. In addition, setting up a valid design in rehabilitation research implies the need to carefully select the variables of interest and operationalize them appropriately. These may be sampled from various domains of patient reported outcomes in terms of, e.g., quality of life and subjective well-being, or from biomedical or socio-economic domains covering outcomes such as frequency of re-hospitalization, survival, health behavior, health care costs, return to work, or others.

9   Summary and Outlook

This chapter presented a brief overview of some major features of cancer rehabilitation. The model of functional health as provided by the ICF served as a background for conceptualizing cancer rehabilitation as a system of coordinated efforts to overcome the functional impairments and activity limitations that have resulted from cancer and its treatment with the aim of restoring functional independence and participation of a patient at the highest possible level. Although countries obviously differ with respect to the way they organize cancer rehabilitation services, they widely share a consensus with respect to the goals of these services. Epidemiologic trends in cancer incidence and prevalence that have contributed to an increase in the importance of cancer rehabilitation thus far were described. It was further pointed out that cancer rehabilitation requires careful individual assessment and in the light of the multifaceted sequelae of cancer and its treatment is probably best provided by a multidisciplinary team. Next, a variety of interventions available to cancer rehabilitation were introduced. Finally, results from evaluation research on the effectiveness of cancer rehabilitation at the level of either single interventions or a rehabilitation program as a whole were discussed. This research suggests meaningful improvements of relevant outcome parameters like quality of life and functional status during the course of rehabilitation and there is also some evidence of cost-effectiveness. However, methodological challenges exist as well, e.g., with respect to the stability of improvements in the patients' quality of life, subjective well-being, and psychological status beyond rehabilitation and with respect to the feasibility of randomization. Nevertheless, future research in cancer rehabilitation will be able to effectively address issues like these and thus will continue to help refine and optimize cancer rehabilitation services. Furthermore, cancer rehabilitation will gain additional importance given the persistence of the epidemiologic trends illustrated in this chapter. Insofar as the utility of cancer rehabilitation programs could further be supported by empirical studies this would once more highlight that cancer rehabilitation serves both the individual patient and society as a whole.

References

Alfano CM, Ganz PA, Rowland JH, Hahn EE (2012) Cancer survivorship and cancer rehabilitation: revitalizing the link. J Clin Oncol 30:904–906. doi:10.1200/JCO.2011.37.1674

Bartsch HH, Weis J, Moser M (2003) Cancer-related fatigue in patients attending oncological rehabilitation programs: prevalence, patterns and predictors. Onkologie 26:51–57

Becker S, Kirchberger I, Cieza A, Berghaus A, Harréus U, Reichel O, Tschiesner U (2010) Content validation of the comprehensive ICF core set for Head and Neck Cancer (HNC): the perspective of psychologists. Psychooncology 19:594–605. doi:10.1002/pon.1608

Bengel J, Wirtz M, Zwingmann C (2008) Diagnostische Verfahren in der Rehabilitation. (Diagnostik für Klinik und Praxis–Band 5). Hogrefe, Göttingen

Bergelt C, Koch U (2002) Rehabilitation bei Tumorpatienten In: Schwarzer R, Jerusalem M, Weber H Gesundheitspsychologie von A–Z, pp. 455–458. Hogrefe, Göttingen

Bornbaum CC, Doyle PC, Skarakis-Doyle E, Theurer JA (2013) A critical exploration of the international classification of functioning, disability, and health (ICF) framework from the perspective of oncology: recommendations for revision. J Multidiscip Healthc 6:75–686. doi: 10.2147/JMDH.S40020

Brach M, Cieza A. Stucki G., Füßl M, Cole A, Ellerin B, Fialka-Moser V, Kostanjsek N, Melvin J (2004) ICF core sets for breast cancer. J Rehabil Med Suppl 44:121–127

Bray F, Jemal A, Grey N, Ferlay J, Forman D (2012) Global cancer transitions according to the human development index (2008–2030): a population-based study. Lancet Oncol 13:790–801. doi:10.1016/S1470-2045(12)70211-5

Cancer Research UK (2011) CancerStats. Cancer World wide. http://www.cancerresearchuk. org/cancer-info/cancerstats/world/the-global-picture/ Accessed 30 Mar 2013

Cancer Research UK (2012) World Cancer fact sheet. World Cancer burden (2008). http://publications.cancerresearchuk.org/downloads/product/CS_FS_WORLD_A4.pdf. Accessed 2 May 2013

Cramp F, Byron-Daniel J (2012) Exercise for the management of cancer-related fatigue in adults. Cochrane Database Syst Rev 11: CD006145. doi:10.1002/14651858.CD006145.pub3

Deutsche Rentenversicherung Bund (2012a) Reha-Bericht 2012. Die medizinische und berufliche Rehabilitation der Rentenversicherung im Licht der Statistik. DRV Bund, Berlin

Deutsche Rentenversicherung Bund (2012b) Reha-Bericht Update 2012. Die medizinische und berufliche Rehabilitation der Rentenversicherung im Licht der Statistik. DRV Bund, Berlin

Deutsches Institut für Medizinische Dokumentation und Information (2005) Internationale Klassifikation der Funktionsfähigkeit. Behinderung und Gesundheit, WHO, Geneva

Edwards AG, Hulbert-Williams N, Neal RD (2008) Psychological interventions for women with metastatic breast cancer. Cochrane Database Syst Rev 16: CD004253. doi: 10.1002/14651858.CD004253.pub3

Faller H, Schuler M, Richard M, Heckl U, Weis J, Küffner R (2013) Effects of psycho-oncologic interventions on emotional distress and quality of life in adult patients with cancer: systematic review and meta-analysis. J Clin Oncol 31(6):782–793. doi:10.1200/JCO.2011.40.8922

Ferlay J, Shin HR, Bray F, Forman D, Mathers C, Parkin DM (2010) Estimates of worldwide burden of cancer in 2008: GLOBOCAN 2008. Int J Cancer 127:2893–2917. doi:10.1002/ijc.25516

Fialka-Moser V, Crevenna R, Korpan M, Quittan M (2003) Cancer rehabilitation. Particularly with aspects on physical impairment. J. Rehabil Med 35:153–162

Gamble GL, Gerber LH, Spill GR, Paul KL (2011) The future of cancer rehabilitation: emerging subspecialty. Am J Phys Med Rehabil 90(5 Suppl 1):S76–S87. doi:10.1097/PHM. 0b013e31820be0d1

Ganz PA, Schag CA, Lee JJ, Sim MS (1992) The CARES: a generic measure of health-related quality of life for patients with cancer. Qual Life Res 1:19–29

Gerber L (2001) Cancer rehabilitation in the future. Cancer 92 4 (Suppl.):975–979

Gerber L, Vargo M, Smith R (2005) Rehabilitation of the cancer patient. In: DeVita V et al (eds) Cancer: principles and pracitce of oncology, 7th edn, pp 3089–3110. Lippincott William, Philadelphia

Gilchrist LS, Galantino ML, Wampler M, Marchese VG, Morris GS, Ness KK (2009) A framework for assessment in oncology rehabilitation. Phys Ther 89:286–306. doi:10.2522/ptj.20070309

Glaessel A, Kirchberger I, Stucki G, Cieza A (2011) Does the comprehensive international classification of functioning, disability and health (ICF) core set for breast cancer capture the problems in functioning treated by physiotherapists in women with breast cancer? Physiotherapy 97:33–46. doi:10.1016/j.physio.2010.08.010

Haaf HG (2005) Ergebnisse zur Wirksamkeit der Rehabilitation. Rehabilitation 44:259–276 (English abstract)

Heim ME, Kunert S, Ozkan I (2001) Effects of inpatient rehabilitation on health-related quality of life in breast cancer patients. Onkologie 24:268–272

Hellbom M, Bergelt C, Bergenmar M, Gijsen B, Loge JH, Rautalahti M, Smaradottir A, Johansen C (2011) Cancer rehabilitation: a nordic and european perspective. Acta Oncol 50:179–186. doi:10.3109/0284186X.2010.533194

Hergert A, Hofreuter K, Melchior H, Morfeld M, Schulz H, Watzke B, Koch U, Bergelt C (2009) Effektivität von Interventionen in der Rehabilitation bei Prostatakarzinompatienten – Ein systematischer Literaturüberblick. Phys Med Rehab Kuror 19:311–325

Holland JC, Breitbart WS, Jacobson PB, Lederberg MS, Loscalzo MJ, McCorkle R (eds) (2010) Psycho-oncology, 2nd edn. Oxford University Press, New York

Koch U, Gundelach C, Tiemann F, Mehnert A (2000) Teilstationäre onkologische Rehabilitation–Ergebnisse eines Modellprojektes. Rehabilitation, 39:363–372 (English abstract)

Koch U, Morfeld M (2004) Weiterentwicklungsmöglichkeiten der ambulanten Rehabilitation in Deutschland. Rehabilitation 43(5):284–295 (English abstract)

Koch U, Weis J (1992) Krebsrehabilitation in der Bundesrepublik Deutschland–eine kritische Betrachtung unter rehabilitationspsychologischer Perspektive. Strahlenther Onkol 168:622–627 (English abstract)

Krüger A, Leibbrand B, Barth J, Berger D, Lehmann C, Koch U, Mehnert A (2009) Verlauf der psychosozialen Belastung und gesundheitsbezogenen Lebensqualität bei Patienten verschiedener Altersgruppen in der onkologischen Rehabilitation. Z Psychosom Med Psychother 55:141–161 (English abstract)

Leib A, Cieza A, Tschiesner U (2012) Perspective of physicians within a multidisciplinary team: content validation of the comprehensive ICF core set for head and neck cancer. Head Neck 34:956–966. doi:10.1002/hed.21844

Meyer T, Gutenbrunner C, Bickenbach J, Cieza A, Melvin J, Stucki G (2011) Towards a conceptual description of rehabilitation as a health strategy. J Rehabil Med 43:765–769. doi: 10.2340/16501977-0865

Mishra SI, Scherer RW, Geigle PM, Berlanstein DR, Topaloglu O, Gotay CC, Snyder C (2012) Exercise interventions on health-related quality of life for cancer survivors. Cochrane Database Syst Rev 8:CD007566. doi:10.1002/14651858.CD007566.pub2

Mpofu E, Oakland T (eds) (2010) Rehabilitation and health assessment: applying ICF guidelines. Springer, New York

Newell SA, Sanson-Fisher RW, Savolainen NJ (2002) Systematic review of psychological therapies for cancer patients: overview and recommendation for future research. J Natl Cancer Inst 94:558–584

NHMCR (2003) Clinical practice guidelines for the psychosocial care of adults with cancer. Australian Government. National Breast Cancer Center. www.nhmrc.gov.au

Oeffinger KC, McCabe MS (2006) Models for delivering survivorship care. J Clin Oncol 24:5117–5124

Puetz TW, Herring MP (2012) Differential effects of exercise on cancer-related fatigue during and following treatment: a meta-analysis. Am J Prev Med 43:e1–e24. doi:10.1016/j.amepre.2012.04.027

Ruppert LM, Stubblefield MD, Stiles J, Passik SD (2010) Rehabilitation medicine in oncology. In: Holland JC, Breitbart WS, Jacobson PB, Lederberg MS, Loscalzo MJ, McCorkle R (eds) Psycho-oncology, 2nd edn. Oxford University Press, New York, pp 460–463

Salz T, Oeffinger KC, McCabe MS, Layne TM, Bach PB (2012) Survivorship care plans in research and practice. CA Cancer J Clin. doi:10.3322/caac.20142

Schag CA, Ganz PA, Heinrich RL (1991) Cancer rehabilitation evaluation system–short form (CARES-SF). A cancer specific rehabilitation and quality of life instrument. Cancer 68:1406–1413

Schwiersch M, Stepien J, Schroeck R (1994) Veraenderungen der Lebensqualitaet von Tumorpatientinnen und -patienten nach stationaerer onkologischer Rehabilitation Die psychosoziale Situation zu Beginn und am Ende eines stationaeren Heilverfahrens sowie ein Jahr danach. Praxis der Klinischen Verhaltensmedizin und Rehabilitation 28:230–240

Spelten ER, Verbeek JH, Uitterhoeve AL, Ansink AC, van der Lelie J, de Reijke TM, Kammeijer M, de Haes JC, Sprangers MA (2003) Cancer, fatigue and the return of patients to work-a prospective cohort study. Eur J Cancer 39:1562–1567

Spence RR, Heesch KC, Eakin EG, Brown WJ (2007) Randomised controlled trial of a supervised exercise rehabilitation program for colorectal cancer survivors immediately after chemotherapy: study protocol. BMC Cancer 7:154

Stout NL, Binkley JM, Schmitz KH, Andrews K, Hayes SC, Campbell KL, McNeely ML, Soballe PW, Berger AM, Cheville AL, Fabian C, Gerber LH, Harris SR, Johansson K, Pusic AL, Prosnitz RG, Smith RA (2012) A prospective surveillance model for rehabilitation for women with breast cancer. Cancer 118:2191–2200. doi:10.1002/cncr.27476

Stubblefield MD, O'Dell MW (eds) (2009) Cancer rehabilitation: principles and practice. Demos Medical Publishing, New York

Teichmann JV (2002) Onkologische Rehabilitation: Evaluation der Effektivität stationärer onkologischer Reha-Maßnahmen. Die Rehabilitation 41:48–52 (English abstract)

Tschiesner U, Linseisen E, Coenen M, Rogers S, Harreus U, Berghaus A, Cieza A (2009) Evaluating sequelae after head and neck cancer from the patient perspective with the help of the international classification of functioning, disability and health. Eur Arch Otorhinolaryngol 266:425–436. doi:10.1007/s00405-008-0764-z

Tschiesner U, Rogers S, Dietz A, Yueh B, Cieza A (2010) Development of ICF core sets for head and neck cancer. Head Neck 32:210–220. doi:10.1002/hed.21172

van Weert E, Hoekstra-Weebers J, Grol B, Otter R, Arendzen HJ, Postema K, Sanderman R, van der Schans C (2005) A multidimensional cancer rehabilitation program for cancer survivors: effectiveness on health-related quality of life. J Psychosom Res 58(6):485–496

van Weert E, Hoekstra-Weebers J, Otter R, Postema K, Sanderman R, van der Schans C (2006) Cancer-related fatigue: predictors and effects of rehabilitation. Oncologist 11:184–196

van Weert E, May AM, Korstjens I, Post WJ, van der Schans CP, van den Borne B, Mesters I, Ros WJ, Hoekstra-Weebers JE (2010) Cancer-related fatigue and rehabilitation: a randomized controlled multicenter trial comparing physical training combined with cognitive-behavioral therapy with physical training only and with no intervention. Phys Ther 90(10):1413–1425. doi:10.2522/ptj.20090212. Epub 2010 Jul 22. Erratum in: Phys Ther. 2010 Dec. 90(12):1906

Weis J, Domann U (2006) Interventionen in der Rehabilitation von Mammakarzinompatientinnen: Eine methodenkritische Uebersicht zum Forschungsstand. Rehabilitation 45:129–142 (English abstract)

Weis J, Moser MT, Bartsch HH (2006) Goal-oriented evaluation of inpatient rehabilitation programs for women with breast cancer (ZESOR–Study). In: Jäckel W, Bengel J, Herdt J (eds) Research in rehabilitation: results of a research network in southwest Germany. Schattauer Verlag, Stuttgart, pp 162–171

WHO (1981) Disability prevention and rehabilitation. Report of the WHO expert committee on disability prevention and rehabilitation. Technical report series 668. WHO, Geneva

WHO (2001) International classification of functioning. Disability and Health, WHO, Geneva

Cancer Survivorship in Adults

Cecilie E. Kiserud, Alv A. Dahl, Jon Håvard Loge and Sophie D. Fosså

Abstract

With the favorable trend regarding survival of cancer in the Western world, there is an increasing focus among patients, clinicians, researchers, and politicians regarding cancer survivors' health and well-being. Their number is rapidly growing and more than 3 % of the adult populations in Western countries have survived cancer for 5 years or more. Cancer survivors are at increased risk for a variety of late effects after treatment, some life-threatening such as secondary cancer and cardiac diseases, others might negatively impact on their daily functioning and quality of life. The latter might include fatigue, anxiety disorders and difficulties returning to work while depression does not seem to be more common among survivors than in the general population. Still, the majority of survivors regain their health and social functioning. The field of cancer survivorship research has been rapidly growing. Models for follow-up care of cancer survivors have been proposed, but how to best integrate the knowledge of the field into clinical practice with adequate follow-up of cancer survivors at risk for developing late effects is still an unsolved question.

C. E. Kiserud (✉) · A. A. Dahl · J. H. Loge · S. D. Fosså
National Resource Center for late effects after Cancer Treatment, Oslo University Hospital, Radiumhospitalet, 4953 Nydalen 0424, Oslo, Norway
e-mail: CKK@ous-hf.no

A. A. Dahl
e-mail: a.a.dahl@ibv.uio.no

J. H. Loge
e-mail: j.h.loge@medisin.uio.no

S. D. Fosså
e-mail: s.d.fossa@medisin.uio.no

U. Goerling (ed.), *Psycho-Oncology*, Recent Results in Cancer Research 197,
DOI: 10.1007/978-3-642-40187-9_8, © Springer-Verlag Berlin Heidelberg 2014

Contents

1   General Aspects.. 104
2   Somatic Late Effects 105
    2.1   Second Cancer... 105
    2.2   Cardiotoxicity 106
    2.3   Gonadal Dysfunction and Infertility... 106
    2.4   Peripheral Neuropathy.. 107
    2.5   Muscle and Skeletal Effects... 107
3   Fatigue 108
4   Anxiety and Depression 109
    4.1   Fear of Recurrence 110
    4.2   Posttraumatic Stress Disorder 110
5   Cognitive Problems 111
6   Sexual Problems 111
7   Work and Economy... 112
8   Marriage Rates.. 113
9   Lifestyle Factors 114
10 Follow-up Care Organization... 114
11 Cancer Survivorship Research 116
References.. 117

1   General Aspects

The number of cancer survivors has been steadily increasing in the Western world during the last decades due to increasing cancer incidence, better diagnostic procedures, and more effective treatment modalities. Today, the relative 5-year survival is 60–65 % for patients diagnosed with cancer (American Cancer Society 2012, Verdecchia et al. 2007). In Norway, cancer survivors alive ≥ 5 years from diagnosis represent 3.3 % of the total population (The Cancer Registry of Norway 2010). For some cancer types such as testicular cancer, breast cancer, and Hodgkin's lymphoma, the 5-year relative survival exceeds 90 %. According to cancer types the most common survivor groups are survivors of female breast, prostate, colorectal, and gynecologic cancer (American Cancer Society 2012).

Cancer survivorship can be defined differently according to time since diagnosis and state of the tumor, and for this chapter we define a cancer survivor as a person who has lived at least 5 year beyond diagnosis and is regarded as tumor-free.

The favorable development as to survival after a cancer diagnosis has been followed by a growing clinical and scientific interest concerning health and quality of life among cancer survivors.

Chemotherapy, radiotherapy, surgery, and hormone therapies are the mainstay of cancer treatment, and they are often combined in various multimodal treatments. Adverse effects may occur during these treatments, and eventually continue for a long time after treatment or become permanent. Other adverse effects have their onset some time after treatment has been terminated, but then continue for a long time. Thus, cancer survivors are at increased risk of various medical and psychosocial complications (Fossa et al. 2008, Fosså and Vassilopoulou et al. 2008). Some late effects might be life-threatening, such as second cancer or cardiovascular disorders, while others such as hypogonadism, infertility, sexual dysfunctions, or chronic fatigue (CF) might have negative impact of the survivors' daily function and quality of life, but do not threaten their lives.

One of the challenges related to studies of late effects is that some late effects like second cancer and cardiovascular diseases typically emerge many years after the termination of treatment. Results of such studies might not completely reflect the risk experienced by patients diagnosed today, since they undergo therapies which have been modified compared to those used 10–20 years ago. Therefore, the studies of late effects by its nature most often lag behind treatment currently given. Concerning new and improved treatments we will have to wait 10–30 years in order to identify their adverse effects. And so the chase for late effects will go on.

Many of the conditions that are described as late effects, like sexual dysfunction, cardiovascular disorders, and fatigue, are also prevalent in the general population. The prevalence of these conditions increase with older age and cancer is primarily a disease of older age since two-third of cancers is diagnosed after 60 years of age.

The goals of survivorship care are twofold: (1) To reduce the risk or cancer recurrence, second cancer and other severe diseases, and adverse effects. (2) To alleviate existing and expected physical and psychological adverse effects. These goals have several challenging implications: (1) To what extent shall cured cancer patients be informed of risks far in the future? (2) How often and how intensively shall survivors be screened for possibly upcoming severe adverse effects? (3) Considering the rapidly growing number of cancer survivors, how shall their health care be organized? To our knowledge there are no countries yet that have found the definite answers to these challenges.

In this chapter we will give an overview of the field of cancer survivorship, including the most important somatic, psychological, and psychosocial late effects and aspects regarding follow-care of cancer survivors and challenges for research in survivorship issues.

2   Somatic Late Effects

Approximately 15 % of cancer survivors will be bothered with treatment-related somatic late effects. An overview of the most important is presented here.

2.1   Second Cancer

Selected groups of cancer survivors are shown to have increased risk for development of a second cancer, which might be related to an iatrogenic effect of the cancer therapy and/or a genetic predisposition. Treatment-related solid second cancers are usually diagnosed at a latency of 10–30 years after radiotherapy, and their development is related to the radiation dose within the target field, but also to scattered irradiation beyond the field borders. A typical example is development of breast cancer after mediastinal irradiation/mantle field irradiation for Hodgkin's lymphoma (Swerdlow et al. 2000) and esophageal cancer after thoracic radiotherapy in women with breast cancer (Morton et al. 2012).

During the last two, decades increasing documentation has emerged that cytotoxic drugs in a dose-dependent manner are carcinogenic leading to an increased risk of leukemia (Travis et al. 1999; Kollmannsberger et al. 1998), but also of solid tumors (Swerdlow et al. 2001, Fung et al. 2013)

The association between second cancer and cytotoxic treatment (radiotherapy, cytostatics) has been one of the strongest arguments for the development of risk-adapted strategies in order to reduce the treatment burden as much as possible, while maintaining the highest possible cure rate.

2.2   Cardiotoxicity

Dependent of their previous treatment long-term cancer survivors may develop asymptomatic or symptomatic left ventricle dysfunction, heart failure, premature coronary atherosclerosis, arrhythmia, or sudden cardiac death, most often due to myocardial infarction (Lenihan et al. 2013). Mediastinal radiotherapy and treatment with certain cytotoxic drugs (antracyclines, trastuzumab) represent well-known cardiotoxic risk factors, with clear dose–effect associations to cardiac dysfunction. Age below 15 years at primary treatment increases the risk. Increased risk of late cardiotoxicity (after 5–30 years) is also reported in breast cancer survivors who have undergone adjuvant cytotoxic treatment (thoracic radiotherapy, systemic cytostatics) (Darby et al. 2013). The European Society of Medical Oncology has recently published recommendations regarding the early detection of cardiotoxicity in patients at risk (Curigliano et al. 2012), but currently there is no international consensus about the optimal procedure for early detection or follow-up of cancer survivors at increased risk of cardiotoxicity.

In addition to a direct cardiac injury due to cytotoxic treatment, the development of metabolic syndrome (overweight, hyperlipidemia, hypertension, hyperglycosuria) represents a risk to the heart. This syndrome is described in long-term testicular (Haugnes et al. 2010, Willemse et al. 2013) and ovarian cancer survivors after cisplatin-based chemotherapy (Liavaag et al. 2009), but is also responsible for the increased risk of cardiac mortality in prostate cancer patients in particular after long-term androgen deprivation therapy (Kenney et al. 2012). Patients at risk should therefore be educated about the importance of a healthy life style (physical activity, healthy diet, no smoking, and moderate use of alcohol).

2.3 Gonadal Dysfunction and Infertility

All surgery, radiotherapy, chemotherapy, and long-term hormone treatment can lead to primary or secondary hypogonadism dependent on whether the damage primarily affects the testicles/ovaries or the pituitary gland/hypothalamus. In addition, the transport of the ovum or the sperm cells may be impeded by fibrosis or stenosis of the ducts because of surgery or radiotherapy.

There are important gender-related differences as to development, prevention, and possible therapy of treatment-related hypogonadism in cancer survivors. After low or intermediate doses of most cytotoxic drugs or after testicular irradiation of less than 2 Gy the sperm cell production can recover as long as spermatogonial stem cells are preserved. The testosterone producing Leydig cells are relatively resistant to chemotherapy and radiotherapy. Severe endocrine hypogonadism is therefore rare after cancer treatment in males. However, clinicians should keep in mind that long-term cancer survivors' testosterone production appears to decrease faster than observed during physiological aging in the male general population.

The situation as to recovery of gonadal function is different in female survivors. At birth the ovaries contain approximately 10 million follicles. This number decreases along with aging up to menopause without replacement of follicles lost each month. After radiotherapy and chemotherapy the loss of follicles is accelerated. As no recovery is possible, female survivors are at risk of premature endocrine and exocrine ovarian failure (menopause before the age of 40).

Treatment of endocrine gonadal failure is based on the application of testosterone or estrogens, however, with important contra-indications in survivors after prostate and breastcancer. Prevention is the best way to limit infertility problems in cancer survivors. Updated guidelines are repeatedly published (Kenney et al. 2012; Metzger et al. 2013). Pretreatment sperm cell cryopreservation has been used for many years in adult male cancer patients, but is problematic in pre-pubertal boys. Pretreatment ovarian or testicular tissue cryoconservation is still experimental, but reimplantation of thawed ovarian tissue has been followed by pregnancies in a few cancer survivors after reimplantation of cryopreserved ovarian tissue. Overall pregnancy rates after adult-onset cancer are decreased by 26 % in male and by 39 % in female cancer patients compared to the general population. After implementation of risk-adapted cancer therapy, this discrepancy has been reduced for selected cancer types during the last three decades (e.g., in testicular cancer survivors or male survivors after Hodgkin's lymphoma) (Stensheim et al. 2011).

2.4 Peripheral Neuropathy

One of the most common late effects (20–30 %) is peripheral neuropathy caused by chemotherapy containing vinca alkaloids, cisplatin, or taxanes (Windebank and Grisold 2008). For some patients the complaints are limited to numbness of soles of the feet, whereas others suffer from pain in the legs that might cause severe sleeping problems. Cisplatin is in addition ototoxic and can lead to tinnitus and hearing loss (Brydøy et al. 2009, Oldenburg et al. 2007). Though the latter toxicity most often is restricted to decibel frequencies of >4000 Hz, severe ototoxicity has a negative impact on a person's social and professional life.

2.5 Muscle and Skeletal Effects

As proliferating cells are particularly sensitive to any cytotoxic treatment, radiotherapy to the skeleton and muscles in young adults can be followed by severe muscle atrophy and retarded growth of bones. The negative impact of the target dose is increased by chemotherapy with radiosensitizing drugs (Actinomycin D, Anthracyclines, Cisplatin) often applied as a part of multimodal therapy.

In breast cancer survivors reduced function of the ipsilateral arm/shoulder, pain and/or lymphoedema have represented frequent complaints, but the incidence of these late effects has been reduced after the introduction of breast conserving surgery and improved radiotherapy techniques (Nesvold et al. 2011)

Osteoporosis related to male and female endocrine hypogonadism may become a problem in all cancer survivors (Lustberg et al. 2012). Prostate cancer and breast cancer survivors are at particular high risk of developing this late effect as complete intermittent or permanent hypogonadism is an important part of their treatment. Today several drugs are available which together with Vitamin D, calcium application and physical activity reduce the risk of osteoporosis by nonhormonal mechanisms (Zoledronic acid, Denosumab).

3 Fatigue

Fatigue is defined as a subjective experience of tiredness, exhaustion, and lack of energy (Radbruch et al. 2008). Formal diagnostic criteria for "cancer-related fatigue" (CRF) as a syndrome were proposed in 1998, but has attracted relatively little attention in the scientific community (Donovan et al. 2013). In this context fatigue is regarded as a symptom.

For most cancer patients, fatigue is experienced as a side-effect during treatment and resolves by recovery from therapy. This can be conceptualized as acute fatigue. However, for some patients, fatigue may persist for years after completed cancer therapy and without any signs of active cancer disease. The term CF, defined as fatigue lasting for 6 months or more or after the stimuli has ended, applies well to such fatigue because the term differentiates between fatigue as part of everyday strains such as acute infections or psychosocial strains and the feeling of being chronically exhausted. Such a distinction is also supported by the fact that fatigue is a very common symptom in the general population (Loge et al. 1998).

The prevalence of fatigue among cancer survivors vary by assessment method, cancer type and definitions, but most prevalence figures vary between 19 and 38 % (Stone and Minton 2008). Survivors of Hodgkin lymphoma and breast cancer are the types most studied. Recent data also indicate that fatigue is common among long-term survivors of cancer in childhood and adolescence (Hamre et al. 2013). Fatigue is therefore probably the commonest late effect across all cancer survivors.

The present knowledge about etiology and mechanisms of fatigue among disease-free cancer survivors is limited (Stone and Minton 2008). It is also unlikely that any single mechanism will be identified because fatigue is multifactorial in origin and is also observed across a variety of noncancer diseases and illnesses. The etiology is therefore best considered as multifactorial, involving both physical and psychological factors. Psychological distress, pain, sleep disturbance, depression, anxiety, inactivity, late medical effects, inflammation, and anemia have all been associated with CRF (Stone and Minton 2008). Except for anemia, all are relevant in relation to CRF among cancer survivors.

Interventions to improve CRF among cancer survivors broadly fall into three categories; drug interventions, exercise interventions, and psychosocial interventions (Stone and Minton 2008). A recent update of a 2008 Cochrane review on drug therapy concluded that psychostimulants are promising but large-scaled randomized controlled trials are warranted (Minton et al. 2010). However, many of the reviewed studies included cancer patients with active disease, and the administration of psychostimulants to disease-free cancer survivors has ethical and legal aspects that need to be clarified. Exercise interventions, mostly consisting of graded aerobic exercise, have slightly to moderate positive effects upon CRF among cancer patients in general (Cramp and Daniel 2008). The strongest effects were observed among cancer survivors, but optimal type, amount and timing of interventions need to be sorted out. Psychosocial interventions include education, coping strategy training, behavioral therapy, cognitive therapy, and supportive therapy. These interventions have slight to moderate effects (Pachman et al. 2012). Education about fatigue, teaching self-care, energy conservation and activity management are easily applied in ordinary clinical contexts. In combination with sleep regulation focusing on night-time sleep, rest without sleeping during daytime, and graded physical exercise, are the best documented interventions that are applicable in ordinary clinical practice.

4   Anxiety and Depression

Longitudinal studies of depression and anxiety after cancer diagnosis suggest that the high early prevalence rates fall slowly over time. The prevalence of depression in long-term cancer survivors was similar to that of healthy controls (Mitchell et al. 2013). The proportion of depressed individuals among spouses of cancer survivors was similar to that of survivors.

Some studies have observed low levels of depression and distress as well as good quality of life (QOL) in long-term cancer survivors. In several studies QOL in long-term cancer survivors is similar to that of the general population (Mykletun et al. 2005).

In contrast, the risk of anxiety disorders is significantly higher among cancer survivors than among healthy controls. Anxiety has also been reported to be as common in spouses as in survivors (Mitchell et al. 2013). In the time frame of 10 years since diagnosis, anxiety shows a more persistent pattern than depression. The distribution of anxiety disorders among cancer survivors did not differ from that of the general population (Greer et al. 2011). In general, presence of anxiety has a negative effect on QOL. The common factor may be distressed (type D) personality, which is the conjoint effect of negative affectivity and social inhibition. The prevalence of type D personality among cancer survivors (19 %) is similar to the general population (13–24 %), but such survivors are at increased risk for impaired QOL and mental health problems (Mols et al. 2012).

4.1   Fear of Recurrence

Recently, more empirical studies have addressed fear of recurrence (Simard et al. 2013). Although defined in various ways, increasing consensus focuses on a fear that cancer could return or progress in the same place or in another part of the body. Various definitions have lead to multiple self-report measures for assessment of fear of recurrence without international recommendations so far (Thewes et al. 2012). This situation may also explain the wide range of prevalence rates reported. According to the review of Simard et al. (Simard et al. 2013) based on 130 papers, across cancer sites, 39–97 % of cancer survivors reported fear of recurrence, 22–87 % reported moderate to high degree, and 0–15 % high degree of such fear. Fear of recurrence seems to remain stable over time, even if the risk of recurrence decreases as time goes on. This finding points to an element of irrationality in fear of recurrence which is common to all kinds of pathological anxiety. The risk of recurrence among long-term testicular cancer survivors is minimal, but still 7 % reported 'very high' and 24 % 'quite a bit' fear of recurrence in our national Norwegian follow-up study (Skaali et al. 2009). This finding has to be considered in the light of the 'focusing illusion' phenomenon which implies considerable exaggeration if people are asked to focus on just one factor concerning their well-being (Kahneman et al. 2006).

4.2   Posttraumatic Stress Disorder

Posttraumatic Stress Disorder (PTSD) is a mental disorder due to exposure to a life-threatening event either personally or as a bystander. Since 1994 "being diagnosed with a life-threatening illness" has been defined as such a potentially traumatic event, and the studies of PTSD among cancer patients have flourished since then. The PTSD symptoms are quite specific with intrusion in the mind of experiences of cancer diagnosis and treatment, and avoidance and hypervigilance in relation to all associations with cancer. The level of PTSD symptoms is regularly high during diagnosis and treatment and then the level gradually tapers off.

Most studies of cancer survivors do not report elevated prevalences of PTSD in cancer survivors compared to the general population. These findings indicate that getting cancer on a group level is not among the most potent traumas in life. However, Smith et al. reported a prevalence of 37 % among survivors of non-Hodgkin lymphomas at a median of 12.9 years after diagnosis, indicating that cancer may be a tougher trauma than expected (Smith et al. 2011). However, in Germany Mehnert and Koch found that 12 % of breast cancer survivors had persistent PTSD (>60 months after diagnosis) (Mehnert and Koch 2008). This prevalence is similar to that observed in the general German female population. Presence of PTSD was associated with younger age, lower level of education, less social support, and progressive disease. These risk factors as well as previous traumas, mental disorders, chemotherapy, and somatic-comorbidity are reported in many studies.

5   Cognitive Problems

Subjective cognitive problems cover cancer patients' complaints concerning memory, concentration, word finding, planning, and doing multiple tasks. A considerable proportion of patients describe such problems when treated with chemotherapy. However, usually these complaints follow the course of anxiety and depression with gradual reduction over time. A minority gets permanent subjective problems. In an American population study, 14 % of cancer patients (brain tumors excluded) reported subjective cognitive complaints versus 8 % among cancer-free controls (Pierre et al. 2011).

Objective evidence for cognitive problems can be documented through neuropsychological tests. Koppelmanns et al. reported considerable neuropsychological deficits in long-term breast cancer survivors compared to cancer-free controls (Koppelmanns et al. 2012). This result has been replicated in several studies with repeated measurements showing long-term neuropsychological deficits particularly after chemotherapy. Functional brain imaging can visualize reduced metabolism in relevant brain areas during neuropsychological testing. For example, de Ruiter et al. showed that long-term breast cancer survivors treated with high-dose chemotherapy 10 years previously, showed significantly less metabolic activation under testing compared to controls (Ruiter et al. 2011).

One problem within this field is the lack of correspondence between subjective complaints and objective findings, which should not be hold against the patient. Another is that cognitive reduction is multifactorial, which makes it difficult to tease out the specific effect of chemotherapy among other factors. For the clinician it is important to keep in mind that cognitive reduction can be a long-term adverse effect after cancer therapy, and that this effect may reduce work ability in particular.

6   Sexual Problems

In this field clinicians should be aware of two facts: (1) Various sexual problems are common in the general population, and information about precancer function is important, not least in order to understand to what extent preexisting problems later on are attributed to cancer. (2) After cancer treatment the optimal aim is to regain the precancer level of sexual function. Cancer hardly improves sexual function, although more openness and emotionality between partners eventually can improve intimacy.

A useful distinction is to separate sexual function in younger and older cancer survivors. Younger survivors are more sexually active, and fertility (see separate section) is still an important issue. Younger survivors concerns mainly survivors of breast and gynecological cancer, lymphomas and other hematological cancers, and sarcomas and testicular cancer. Finally, a general complaint is the lack of communication about sexuality between survivors and both clinicians and general practitioners.

There are few studies of sexuality in long-term survivors. A recent review did not specify time of survival and was thereby less helpful (Bober and Varela 2012). The same critique can be raised toward a review of studies in gynecological cancer survivors (Abbott-Anderson and Kwekkeboom 2012).

Among younger survivors the issue of sexual function in long-term testicular cancer survivors has been debated, however the controlled study with the largest sample, hardly observed significant differences from population-based controls (Dahl et al. 2007). In contrast, long-term male survivors of lymphomas had significantly poorer sexual function than such controls (Kiserud et al. 2009). Young female breast cancer patients often experience long-term lack of sexual interest. The attitude of their partners toward their body and femininity is very important for their sexual well-being. Premature menopause and hormone therapy also is of considerable importance, but less so for long-term survivors.

Most of the same issues are relevant for older breast cancer survivors. In gynecological cancer survivors lack of interest, vaginal dryness, and pains during intercourse are common complaints. Colorectal cancer is followed by high rates of sexual dysfunctions in both males and females at a mean of 4 years since diagnosis (Ousten et al. 2012). Both radical prostatectomy and radiotherapy for prostate cancer as well as adjuvant hormone treatment are mostly followed by severe long-term erectile dysfunction, and sexual recovery is seldom achieved (Wittmann et al. 2009).

7   Work and Economy

Work ability is a concept which covers a person's ability to take part in ordinary work life and has three components: physical, mental, and social ability (van den Berg et al. 2009). Cancer most often infers a weakening of the physical work ability that can be temporary or permanent. However, cancer can also affect the mental and social work ability. In the Nordic countries over 80 % of men and women are active in work life, the big difference being that most of the men, but only half of the women hold full-time work. For those at work, when they get their cancer diagnosis, *return to work* is the first important issue. Within 2 years after diagnosis approximately 60 % (range 30–93 %) reenter work life (Taskila et al. 2007). Based on 26 studies, de Boer et al. reported a general unemployment rate of 33.8 % in cancer patients compared to 15.2 % in controls (RR 1.37, 95 %CI 1.21–1.55) (Boer et al. 2009).

These findings point not only to return to work, but also to the problem of *staying at work* for cancer survivors. Several studies have examined the *problems of cancer survivors at the workplace*. Most studies concern women with breast cancer who report that cognitive problems, hot flashes, and arm-shoulder morbidity reduced their work productivity. Pain in general and fatigue were common problems for survivors of both genders. In patients treated with surgery for prostate cancer physical tasks like lifting and stooping, can be associated with socially incapacitating urinary leakage, but cognitive problems at work were also common in men treated for prostate cancer. Difficulties of coping with previous job demands and expectation of employers and colleagues were common. Interestingly, over-protectiveness from colleagues was also commonly reported as a problem. Follow-up studies concerning *stability in work life over time* are uncommon so far. In our unpublished studies of testicular cancer survivors and survivors of breast cancer stage I, we observed that long-term stability in work life in these groups of cancer survivors which have very good prognosis, was similar to that of the general population.

When work ability is permanently reduced, persons have to leave the work force and go on to disability pension. Compared to matched controls without cancer, survivors have a significantly higher rate of disability pension (Carlsen et al. 2008, Hauglann et al. 2012) Compared to being at work, disability pension implies an income reduction, and several studies have shown that cancer survivors have permanently lower income compared to matched controls without cancer. However, due to generous welfare compensations in Norway the income reduction for cancer survivors is small compared to the general population (Syse and Tønnessen 2012).

Cancer survivors as a group display a reduction in working hours and >10 % decline in overall earnings. There are differences across diagnoses with survivors of lymphomas, lung, brain, bone, colorectal, and head-and neck cancer being mostly affected by decline in earnings. Other factors negatively effecting upon earnings are low level of education, lower social support, chemotherapy, self-employment, shorter tenure in the job, and part-time work (Mehnert 2011).

8 Marriage Rates

Marriage rate is a relevant outcome among survivors of cancers hitting in childhood, adolescence, and early adulthood. Generally, negative effects upon marriage rates are depending upon several disease-treatment and host-related factors including late medical effects and their interplay. Further, cultural and societal differences might modify or exaggerate the effects implying that findings from one country not necessarily are transferrable to other countries with for example different school or health care systems (Syse and Geller 2011).

A registry-based study from Norway including all Norwegian cancer survivors 17–44 years old diagnosed in the period 1974–2001, found the marriage rates of survivors of most types of cancer to be similar to the age-matched Norwegian population as a whole. Some subgroups such as women with brain and breast cancer had lower marriage rates than their cancer-free counterparts (Syse 2008).

9 Lifestyle Factors

Lifestyle factors are important for cancer survivors since they represent risk factors for relapse of the primary cancer, development of secondary cancer, and development of comorbid diseases, like diabetes, which reduce the health status and quality of life of the survivors.

The lifestyle factors are well-known: smoking, diet, low physical activity, and high alcohol consumption. Although the severe consequences of unhealthy lifestyle are well-known, permanent lifestyle changes have proved difficult to implement by health campaigns or other types of mass influence. Getting cancer has been considered a "teachable moment" for life style change, but even rather intensive long-term interventions report only moderate success.

Compared to men in the general population, a higher proportion of testicular cancer survivors are daily smokers (Thorsen ct al. 2005).

Although regular alcohol intake is associated with increased risk for many types of cancer, the relation of such a habit with cancer recurrence and morbidity is unclear. However, the risk for development of additional comorbid somatic diseases is considerable.

Obesity increases the risk of cancer recurrence and mortality, particularly in survivors of breast and prostate cancers (Ligibel 2012). However, weight gain in the survivorship period does not represent a significantly increased risk for these outcomes, and weight loss does not seem to reduce the risk. However, weight loss is important for physical function and reduces the risk for lifestyle diseases like diabetes or hypertension. Among six prospective cohort studies, five have reported a decreased risk of cancer recurrence and related death if the survivors engage in modest levels of physical activity. The documentation is most convincing for survivors of breast, colon and prostate cancer, and concerns walking for 3 h a week at an average pace.

10 Follow-up Care Organization

Follow-up practices for long-term cancer survivors are probably suboptimal in most countries both regarding content and organization. Specialized late-effects clinics have been established in some countries and most of them provide care for survivors of childhood cancers. However, the evidence base for the effects of different models is presently weak (Earle and Ganz 2012). For providers, the challenge is to develop and institute care models that address the needs of the fast growing population of survivors. To our knowledge, the only European national initiative has been launched in Great Britain, the National Cancer Survivorship Initiative (http://www.ncsi.org.uk/). In the United States, both the American Cancer Society and the National Cancer Institute are engaged in developing cancer survivorship care. Due to differences in cultures, resources, and structure of health care systems, models found to be effective in one setting are not necessarily optimal in other settings.

Follow-up of cancer survivors includes three distinct parties: the specialist with expertise of the disease, treatment and risk for late effects; the Primary Care Physician (PCP) with specific knowledge of their patients but often not updated on their risks for late effects; and finally the patient with his/her level of knowledge, attitudes and behavior. Follow-up care might theoretically be delivered by the specialist, the PCP or combinations of the two (shared care). A fourth option is to give the survivor the full responsibility without involving the health care system unless the survivor asks for it.

Follow-up by the treating oncologist for all cancer survivors is not feasible due to lack of manpower and resources in general. Further, not all survivors are in need of specialized follow-up care, and the National Cancer Survivorship Initiative has estimated that about 75 % of all survivors can manage their health themselves with support from the primary health care system (http://www.ncsi.org.uk/). On this background, the concept of risk-based care has been launched and includes development of a systematic plan for prevention and surveillance based on risks associated with the cancer therapy, genetic predispositions, the survivors' lifestyle and comorbidities (Oeffinger and McCab 2006).

For the cancer survivor to be able to make the optimal decisions regarding own present and future health, they need information regarding the long-term health risks they face and how to best handle them. The literature indicates that today's cancer survivors are not aware of their risks for later adverse health events (Kadan-Lottick et al. 2002; Hess et al. 2011). These findings might not only relate to lacking information per se. We must also assume that the survivors have an ambivalent wish for information about future health risks.

Survivorship care plans have been proposed as a means to operationalize the recommendations regarding follow-up care. The idea is that a comprehensive care summary and follow-up plan is written by the principal provider of the oncology care. However, a recent randomized trial could not demonstrate positive effects of such plans among survivors of breast cancer (Grunfeld et al. 2011).

Thus, the present status is that organization and content of follow-up care is still under development. As stated by Earle and Ganz, in this setting it is timely not to let the perfect be the enemy of the good (Earle and Ganz 2012).

11   Cancer Survivorship Research

With the shift from cancer having a poor prognosis to being curable diseases, research questions assessing late effects, who are at particular risk of developing them, how can they best be prevented and managed and how does having had cancer impact upon the living conditions of the survivors, became increasingly relevant as the number of survivors rapidly increased (Rowland et al. 2013).

At the start of cancer survivorship research in the 1970s, survivors of cancers that had recently become curable, that hit early in life and the survivors had a long life expectancy after cure such as childhood cancers, testicular cancers, and Hodgkin's lymphoma, first attracted the researchers' attention. The research field has later rapidly expanded, and by year 2011 nearly 17,500 citations related to cancer survivorship science were identified (Rowland et al. 2013). The rapid expansion includes studies of new groups of survivors and broadening of the research field to include not only quantity of life but also the survivors' quality of life. Noteworthy is the finding that late medical effects continue to emerge decades after end of treatment making continuous surveillance and research on their mechanisms, prevention and treatment even more relevant now than 40 years ago. In conjunction with the expansion of molecular biology, research on the mechanisms of late effects has greatly advanced from year 2000 onward. In the same period, models for providing health care to the survivors and their cost-effectiveness have emerged as a new field of great relevance for the survivors themselves but also for health administrators and health authorities.

Representative national or regional cancer registries or not available in all countries, but when they are, they provide unique opportunities for studying unselected cohorts of survivors. Some research groups have studied survivors previously included in clinical trials. As opposed to registry data, clinical trials usually provide a broad range of variables for characterization of the exposure— i.e., the disease and treatment, and the host at start of treatment. A limitation of using participants form previous clinical trials is the very low rate of cancer patients being included in trials, which infers that the study subjects are highly selected and the findings will have limited external validity. Observational studies by postal questionnaires have probably been the most frequently used design. Questionnaires specifically developed for cancer survivors have been developed and tested (Pearce et al. 2008). Generic questionnaires, disease-specific questionnaires, or questionnaires specifically developed for cancer survivors have been used. The generic questionnaires allow for comparisons with other populations including the general population but lack cancer-specific content. The cancer-specific questionnaires often include content of particular relevance for patients receiving treatment but such content might be less relevant after treatment and when the patient is cured. Cancer survivorship-specific questionnaires such as the Impact of Cancer (IOC) scale (Zebrack et al. 2006) addresses important aspects of survivorship such as personal growth, but has limitations regarding comparisons with populations not affected by cancer. The terms health-related quality of life (HRQOL) and quality of life have been used interchangeably although most studies have used HRQOL-measures (Rowland 2007).

Some important challenges of particular relevance for cancer survivorship research need to be pointed out. One is to define who is a cancer survivor. A second challenge is to identify the survivors 10–20–30 years after end of treatment. Legislations, the structure of the health care system and social mobility all effect upon the possibility to identify the survivors. For example, in Norway due to a unique personal identity number, a national uniform health care system and relatively low social mobility, we have been able to identify nearly all survivors of specific cancers more than 25–30 years after end of treatment. A third important challenge is how to control for age-related health effects when for example studying adult survivors in their 50s and 60s who were treated as children. Choosing an optimal control group is therefore critical and needs careful consideration. A fourth challenge is to have access to data that allows for detailed description of the exposure and the patient at time of exposure. Most studies till now have been cross-sectional and data on the exposure and the host at time of exposure are often not available or very limited. Cross-sectionals designs limit the possibility to draw inferences about causality. Fifthly, funding of research is a challenge in many countries exaggerated by the present financial crisis. Finally, the diversity of end-points, especially patient-reported, hinders comparisons of findings across studies.

References

Abbott-Anderson K, Kwekkeboom KL (2012) A systematic review of sexual concerns reported by gynecological cancer survivors. Gynecol Oncol 124:477–489

American Cancer Society (2012) Cancer Treatment and Survivorship Facts and Figures 2012–2013

Bober SL, Varela VS (2012) Sexuality in adult cancer survivors: challenges and intervention. J Clin Oncol 30:3712–3719

Brydøy M, Oldenburg J, Klepp O et al (2009) Observational study of prevalence of long-term Raynaud-like phenomena and neurological side effects in testicular cancer survivors. J Natl Cancer Inst 101:1682–1695

Carlsen K, Dalton SO, Frederiksen K et al (2008) Cancer and the risk for taking early retirement pension. Scand J Publ Health 36:117–125

Cramp F, Daniel J (2008) Exercise for the management of cancer-related fatigue in adults. Cochrane Database Syst Rev 2:CD006145. doi: 10.1002/14651858.CD006145.pub2

Curigliano G, Cardinale D, Suter T et al (2012) Cardiovascular toxicity induced by chemotherapy, targeted agents and radiotherapy: ESMO clinical practice guidelines. Ann Oncol 23:155–1662

Dahl AA, Bremnes R, Dahl O, Klepp et al (2007) Is the sexual function compromised in long-term testicular cancer survivors? Eur Urol 52:1438–1447

Darby SC, Ewertz M, McGale P et al (2013) Risk of ischemic heart disease in women after radiotherapy for breast cancer. N Engl J Med 368:987–998

de Boer AGEM, Taskila T, Ojajärvi A et al (2009) Cancer survivors and unemployment—a meta-analysis and meta-regression. JAMA 301:753–762

de Ruiter MB, Reneman L, Boogerd W et al (2011) Cerebral hyporesponsiveness and cognitive impairment 10 years after chemotherapy for breast cancer. Hum Brain Map 32:1209–1216

Den Ousten BL, Traa MJ, Thong MSY et al (2012) Higher prevalence of sexual dysfunction in colon and rectal cancer survivors compared with the normative population: a population-based study. Eur J Cancer 48:3161–3170

Donovan KA, McGinty HL, Jacobsen PB (2013) A systematic review of research using the diagnostic criteria for cancer-related fatigue. Psychooncology 22:737–744

Earle CC, Ganz PA (2012) Cancer survivorship care: don't let the perfect be the enemy of the good. J Clin Oncol 30:3764–3768

Fossa SD, Loge JH, Dahl AA (2008) Long-term survivorship after cancer: how far have we come? Ann Oncol S5:25–29

Fosså S, Vassilopoulou-Sellin R, Dahl A (2008) Long term physical sequelae after adult-onset cancer. J Canc Survivorship 2:3–11

Fung C, Fosså SD, Milano MT et al (2013) Solid tumors following chemotherapy or surgery for testicular nonseminoma: A population-based study of 12,691 patients. J Clin Oncol (in press)

Greer JA, Solis JM, Temel JS et al (2011) Anxiety disorders in long-term survivors of adult cancers. Psychosom 52:417–423

Grunfeld E, Julian JA, Pond G et al (2011) Evaluating survivorship care plans: results of a randomized, clinical trial of patients with breast cancer. J Clin Oncol 29:4755–4762

Hamre H, Zeller B, Kanellopoulos A et al (2013) High prevalence of chronic fatigue in adult long-term survivors of acute lymphoblastic leukemia and lymphoma during childhood and adolescence. J Adolesc Young Adult Oncol 2:2–9

Hauglann B, Benth JS, Fosså SD et al (2012) A cohort study of permanently reduced work ability in breast cancer patients. J Cancer Surviv 6:345–356

Haugnes HS, Wethal T, Aass N et al (2010) Cardiovascular risk factors and morbidity in long-term survivors of testicular cancer: a 20-year follow-up study. J Clin Oncol 28:4649–4657

Hess SL, Johannsdottir IM, Hamre H et al (2011) Adult survivors of childhood malignant lymphoma are not aware of their risk of late effects. Acta Oncol 50:653–659

Jean Pierre P, Winters PC, Ahles TA et al (2011) Prevalence of self-reported memory problems in adult cancer survivors: a national cross-sectional study. J Oncol Pract 8:30–34

Kadan-Lottick NS, Robison LL, Gurney JG et al (2002) Childhood cancer survivors' knowledge about their past diagnosis and treatment: childhood cancer survivor study. JAMA 287:1832–1839

Kahneman D, Krueger AB, Schkade D et al (2006) Would you be happier if you were richer? A focusing illusion. Science 312:1908–1910

Kenney LB, Cohen LE, Shnorhavorian M et al (2012) Male reproductive health after childhood, adolescent, and young adult cancers: a report from the Children's Oncology Group. J Clin Oncol 30:3408–3416

Kiserud CE, Schover LR, Dahl AA et. (2009) Do male lymphoma survivors have impaired sexual function? J Clin Oncol 27: 6019–6026

Kollmannsberger C, Beyer J, Droz JP et al (1998) Secondary leukemia following high cumulative doses of etoposide in patients treated for advanced germ cell tumors. J Clin Oncol 16:3386–3391

Koppelmanns V, de Ruiter MB, van der Lijn F et al (2012) Global and focal brain volume in long-term breast cancer survivors exposed to adjuvant chemotherapy. Breast Cancer Res Treat 132:1099–1106

Lenihan D, Oliva S, Chow EJ et al (2013) Cardiac toxicity in cancer survivors. Cancer 119:2131–2142

Liavaag AH, Tonstad S, Pripp AH et al (2009) Prevalence and determinants of metabolic syndrome and elevated Framingham risk score in epithelial ovarian cancer survivors: a controlled observational study. Int J Gynecol Cancer 19:634–640

Ligibel J (2012) Lifestyle factors in cancer survivorship. J Clin Oncol 30:3697–3704

Loge JH, Ekeberg Ø, Kaasa S (1998) Fatigue in the general Norwegian population—normative data and associations. J Psychosom Res 45:53–65

Lustberg MB, Reinbolt RE, Shapiro CL (2012) Bone health in adult cancer survivorship. J Clin Oncol 30:3665–3674

Metzger ML, Meacham LR, Patterson B et al (2013) Female reproductive health after childhood, adolescent, and young adult cancers: guidelines for the assessment and management of female reproductive complications. J Clin Oncol 31:1239–1247

Mehnert A, Koch U (2008) Psychological comorbidity and health-related quality of life and its association with awareness, utilization, and need for psychosocial support in a cancer register-based sample of long-term breast cancer survivors. J Psychosom Res 64:383–391

Mehnert A (2011) Employment and work-related issues in cancer survivors. Critical Rev Oncol/Hematol 77:109–130

Minton O, Richardson A, Sharpe M et al (2010) Drug therapy for the management of cancer-related fatigue. Cochrane Database Syst Rev. 7:CD006704

Mitchell AJ, Ferguson DW, Paul J et al (2013) Depression and anxiety in long-term cancer survivors compared with spouses and healthy controls. Lancet Oncol. doi: 10.1016.S1470-2045(13)70244-4

Mols F, Thong MSY, van de Poll-Franse L et al (2012) Type D (distressed) personality is associated with poor quality of life and mental health among 3080 cancer survivors. J Affect Dis 136:26–34

Morton LM, Gilbert ES, Hall P et al (2012) Risk of treatment-related esophageal cancer among breast cancer survivors. Ann Oncol 23:3081–3091

Mykletun A, Dahl AA, Haaland CF et al (2005) Side effects and cancer-related stress determine quality of life in long-term survivors of testicular cancer. J Clin Oncol 23:3061–3068

Nesvold IL, Reinertsen KV, Fosså SD et al (2011) The relation between arm/shoulder problems and quality of life in breast cancer survivors: a cross-sectional and longitudinal study. J Canc Surviv 5:62–72

Oeffinger KC, McCab MS (2006) Models for delivering survivorship care. J Clin Oncol 24:5117–5124

Oldenburg J, Kraggerud SM, Cvancarova M et al (2007) Cisplatin-induced long-term hearing impairment is associated with specific glutathione s-transferase genotypes in testicular cancer survivors. J Clin Oncol 25:708–714

Pachman DR, Barton DL, Swetz KM et al (2012) Troublesome symptoms in cancer survivors: fatigue, insomnia, neuropathy, and pain. J Clin Oncol 30:3687–3696

Pearce NJ, Sanson-Fisher R, Campbell HS (2008) Measuring quality of life in cancer survivors: a methodological review of existing scales. Psychooncology 17:629–640

Radbruch L, Strasser F, Elsner F et al (2008) Fatigue in palliative care patients-an EAPC approach. Palliat Med 22:13–32

Rowland JH (2007). Survivorship research: past, present and future. In: Ganz PA (ed) Cancer survivorship today and tomorrow. Springer, New York, pp 28–42

Rowland JH, Kent EE, Forsythe LP et al. (2013) Cancer survivorship research in Europe and the United States: where have we been, where are we going, and what can we learn from each other? Cancer 119(S11):2094–2108

Simard S, Thewes B, Humphris G et al (2013) Fear of cancer recurrence in adult cancer survivors. J Cancer Surviv. doi:10.1007/s11764-013-0272-z

Skaali T, Fosså SD, Bremnes R et al (2009) Fear of recurrence in long-term testicular cancer survivors. Psychooncology 18:580–588

Smith SK, Zimmerman S, Williams et al (2011) Post-traumatic stress symptoms in long-term non-Hodgkin's lymphoma survivors. Does time heal? J Clin Oncol 29:4526–4533

Stensheim H, Cvancarova M, Møller B et al (2011) Pregnancy after adolescent and adult cancer: a population-based matched cohort study. Int J Cancer 129:1225–1236

Stone PC, Minton O (2008) Cancer-related fatigue. Eur J Canc 44:1097–1104

Swerdlow AJ, Barber JA, Hudson GV et al (2000) Risk of second malignancy after Hodgkin's disease in a collaborative British cohort: the relation to age at treatment. J Clin Oncol 18:498–509

Swerdlow AJ, Schoemaker MJ, Allerton R et al (2001) Lung cancer after Hodgkin's disease: a nested case-control study of the relation to treatment. J Clin Oncol 19:1610–1618

Syse A (2008) Does cancer affect marriage rates? J Cancer Surviv 2:205–214

Syse A, Geller B (2011) A cross-cultural perspective on challenges facing comparative cancer survivorship research. J Cancer Epidemiol 2011:689025. doi:10.1155/2011/689025

Syse A, Tønnessen M (2012) Cancer's unequal impact on incomes in Norway. Acta Oncol 51:480–489

Taskila T, Martikainen R, Hietanen P et al (2007) Comparative study of work ability between cancer survivors and their referents. Eur J Cancer 43:914–920

The Cancer Registry of Norway (2010) Cancer in Norway 2010

Thewes B, Butow P, Zachariae R et al (2012) Fear of cancer recurrence: a systematic literature review of self-report measures. Psycho-Oncol 21:571–587

Thorsen L, Nystad W, Stigum H et al (2005) The association between self-reported physical activity and prevalence of depression and anxiety disorder in long-term survivors of testicular cancer and men in a general population sample. Support Care Cancer 13:637–646

Travis LB, Holowaty EJ, Bergfeldt K et al (1999) Risk of leukemia after platinum-based chemotherapy for ovarian cancer. N Engl J Med 340:351–357

van den Berg TIJ, Elders LAM, de Zwart BCH et al (2009) The effects of work-related factors on the work ability index: a systematic review. Occup Environ Med 66:211–220

Verdecchia A, Francisci S, Brenner H et al (2007) Recent cancer survival in Europe: a 2000–2002 period analysis of EUROCARE-4 data. Lancet Oncol 8:784–796

Willemse PM, Burggraaf J, Hamdy NA et al (2013) Prevalence of the metabolic syndrome and cardiovascular disease risk in chemotherapy-treated testicular germ cell tumour survivors. Br J Cancer 109(1):295–296 (in press)

Windebank AJ, Grisold W (2008) Chemotherapy-induced neuropathy. J Peripher Nerv Syst 13:27–46

Wittmann D, Northhouse L, Foley S et al (2009) The psychosocial aspects of sexual recovery after prostate cancer treatment. Int J Impotence Res 21:99–106

Zebrack BJ, Ganz PA, Bernaards CA et al (2006) Assessing the impact of cancer: development of a new instrument for long-term survivors. Psychooncology 15:407–421

Psycho-Oncological Interventions and Psychotherapy in the Oncology Setting

Mirjam de Vries and Friedrich Stiefel

Abstract

A person who faces the diagnosis of cancer is subjected to changes within his body, but also with regard to his view of himself and his social relationships. Cancer-related psychological distress occurs frequently and has been reported to have different prevalence according to cancer type and stage of disease. Psychological disorders are known to be underdiagnosed and thus undertreated in the oncology setting, since clinicians might miss the symptoms of psychological distress, misinterpret them, or lack the time and resources to respond adequately. The main psychiatric disturbances observed in patients with cancer are adjustment disorders and affective disorders (anxiety and depression), which in the majority of patients are due to stressors related to the disease and pre-existing psychological vulnerabilities; however, they might also be a direct consequence of biological causes either resulting from treatment side effects or from modifications induced by the cancer. This chapter aims to provide theoretical and practical information concerning psycho-oncological approaches, complemented by some reflexions on their clinical and scientific evidence, focussing essentially on verbal psychological interventions and especially on psychotherapy in patients with cancer.

M. de Vries
Institut Universitaire de Psychothérapie, Département de Psychiatrie, Centre hospitalier universitaire vaudois, Avenue de Morges 10, 1004, Lausanne, Switzerland

F. Stiefel (⊠)
Service de Psychiatrie de Liaision, Département de Psychiatrie, Centre hospitalier universitaire vaudois, Rue du Bugnon 21, 1011, Lausanne, Switzerland
e-mail: Frederic.stiefel@chuv.ch

U. Goerling (ed.), *Psycho-Oncology*, Recent Results in Cancer Research 197,
DOI: 10.1007/978-3-642-40187-9_9, © Springer-Verlag Berlin Heidelberg 2014

Contents

1 Introduction.. 122
2 Psychological Challenges for Patients Facing Cancer and Its Treatment........................ 123
3 Psychological Interventions.. 124
   3.1 Psychoeducation 124
   3.2 Psychological Support.. 124
   3.3 Psychotherapy.. 124
4 Outcome of Psycho-Oncological Interventions... 130
5 Conclusions.. 130
References... 131

1 Introduction

A person who faces the diagnosis of cancer is subjected to changes within his body, but also with regard to his view of himself and his social relationships. Since each individual reacts differently when facing such a life-threatening event, the psychological responses should not be considered as «adequate» or «inadequate» but rather as whether the response is adaptive or an expression of psychological disturbances. Cancer-related psychological distress occurs frequently: for example, prevalence of major depression is estimated to occur in 10–25 %, of depressive symptoms in 21–58 % (Massie 2004; Mitchell et al. 2011; Pirl 2004), and of pathological demoralization in 14 % (Kissane et al. 2004a, b) of patients with cancer. Furthermore, anxiety disorders were reported in 15–28 % of cancer patients (Kerrihard et al. 1999), and a recent meta-analysis showed that 38.2 % of them suffered from any type of emotional disorders (Mitchel et al. 2011), a finding which is confirmed by a large prevalence study which identified 35.1 % to suffer from distress at a clinical level (Zabora et al. 2001). Psychological distress has been reported to have different prevalence according to cancer site: it was found to be highest in pancreatic (56.7 %), lung (43.4 %), and brain cancer (42.7 %), and lower in gynecological (29.6 %), prostate (30.5 %), and colon cancer (31.6 %) (Zabora et al. 2001). Also patients with advanced stages may be more vulnerable to psychological distress, especially when taking into account acute confusional states (Massie 2004; Razavi and Stiefel 1994); however, some research, for example in breast cancer, suggests that stage of cancer does not influence prevalence of psychological distress (Kissane et al. 2004a, b).

Psychological disorders are known to be underdiagnosed and thus undertreated in the oncology setting (Razavi and Stiefel 1994), since clinicians might miss the symptoms of psychological distress, misinterpret them or lack the time and resources to respond adequately.

This chapter aims to provide theoretical and practical information concerning psycho-oncological approaches, complemented by some reflections on their clinical and scientific evidence, focusing essentially on verbal psychological interventions, and especially on psychotherapy in patients with cancer.

2   Psychological Challenges for Patients Facing Cancer and Its Treatment

The main psychiatric disturbances observed in patients with cancer are adjustment disorders and affective disorders (anxiety and depression), which in the majority of patients are due to stressors related to the disease and pre-existing psychological vulnerabilities; however, they might also be a direct consequence of biological causes either resulting from treatment side effects or from modifications induced by the cancer (e.g., treatment with interferon or radiation therapy, brain metastases, hypercalcemia, paraneoplastic syndroms, hypothyreosis) (Razavi and Stiefel 1994).

Therefore, treatment of psychological distress calls for a careful evaluation in order to determine the most appropriate intervention, which might be to focus on biological, psychological, psychopharmacological or combined causal factors. In the following, we will only focus on distress for which psychological interventions are appropriate and beneficial.

From the moment of the diagnosis, the patient is confronted with a new situation that he will need to understand, shape, and accept and which will modify his perception of himself, his interpersonal relationships, and his sense of belonging to a group: he might reflect on his past and will definitely have to adjust to the present and adapt his plans for the future. Pre-existing self-image, quality of interpersonal relationships, and sense of belonging are therefore factors that can either contribute to the protection of the individual against stress and emotional difficulties or they might be a source of increased vulnerability.

Adjustment to cancer is associated with six distinct hurdles, as defined by Faulkner and Maguire (1994): (1) managing uncertainty about the future, (2) searching for meaning, (3) dealing with loss of control, (4) having a need for openness, (5) emotional, and (6) medical support. Failing to deal with these hurdles might lead to psychosocial difficulties. Psychological interventions are often initiated in order to help the patient with these issues so as to help him to cope and adjust to the disease, and have been demonstrated to have a positive effect on distress, anxiety, and depression (Devine and Westlake 1995; Meyer and Mark 1995; Sheard and Maguire 1999).

While the spectrum of psycho-oncological interventions is large, from psychopharmacological treatments, relaxation and music-therapy to psychotherapy, we will concentrate on the verbal psychological interventions and focus on psychotherapy for patients with cancer.

3   Psychological Interventions

3.1   Psychoeducation

Psychoeducation refers to the education offered by a professional to a patient about a mental or physical condition that causes psychological stress. By learning about his condition the patient is thought to feel more in control, which might help to reduce psychological distress.

3.2   Psychological Support

Psychological support knows many definitions and covers approaches from individual psychological support interventions (Hellbom et al. 1998), single techniques derived from psychotherapies, such as relaxation or structured problem-solving, to community or peer support services, and range from one to several sessions. The aims of supportive interventions might be to contribute to alleviate worries of the patient, to increase his perception of mastering the situation, to help him to regulate stress, or to facilitate his participation in the treatment. Psychological support might be presented by health personal or other persons, since its use is generally not regulated or controlled by training institutes or licensing bodies.

3.3   Psychotherapy

Psychotherapy has been defined by Frank (1988) as the relief of distress or disability in one person by another, using an approach based on a particular theory or paradigm, with the requirement that the agent performing the therapy has had training. Franck and Frank (1991) identified four broad dimensions shared by all therapeutic approaches: (i) a relationship in which the patient considers that the therapist is competent and cares about his state; (ii) a setting which is defined as a place of healing; (iii) a rationale which explains the patient's suffering and how it can be overcome; (iv) a set of procedures requiring active participation of the patient and the therapist and of which both believe to be means of restoring the patient's health.

These general dimensions allow the inclusion of all psychotherapeutic interventions, but they lack the specificity to identify an included approach as a psychotherapeutic intervention. Wampold (2001) and Lambert and Ogles (2004) also underline the necessity that psychotherapy is a professional activity or service that implies a certain level of skills, which have to be formally recognized by training institutes and licensing bodies, and anchored in a psychological theory; in addition psychotherapeutic treatment should be supported by scientific evidence and provided by mental health specialists, who undergo training and who benefit from regular supervision and continuous postgraduate education. In many countries, psychotherapeutic treatments can therefore only be provided by certified psychiatrists and psychologists.

In the following, we will present and discuss the three most widely used psychotherapeutic approaches: psychodynamic, systemic, and cognitive behavioral psychotherapy. These approaches have a long history of theoretical and conceptual development and are widely utilized in psychiatric and somatic settings, including oncology. Some of them have gained an important body of evidence confirming their effectiveness and all provide specialized and certified training programs and allow a large clinical application. Finally, the important movement of psychotherapy integration will also be discussed.

3.3.1 Psychodynamic Psychotherapy

Psychodynamic psychotherapies are derived from Freud's work, object relation theory elaborated by Klein and Winnicott and self-psychology based on Sullivan's interpersonal psychotherapy (Lewin 2005). Psychodynamic techniques are intended to develop self-understanding and insight into recurrent problems. In the therapeutic process, symptoms and interpersonal difficulties are identified, analyzed, and interpreted based on the assumption that the subsequent insight and the experiences in the therapeutic relationship can be transferred to «the world outside the therapeutic setting» (Kaplan and Sadock 1998).

Psychodynamic psychotherapies rely on key theoretical concepts, such as (i) the existence of an unconscious, which influences our thoughts, emotions, and behaviors; (ii) the impact of early development on later stages of life; (iii) the organization of the psyche by the ego, which has the capacity to reason and to anticipate, the id, which is a source of sexual and aggressive drives, and the superego, which contains theses drives by a «guilty conscience»; (iv) the protection of the individuals' equilibrium by (unconscious) defense mechanisms, such as rationalization, projection, or denial, which are triggered by threatening emotions or thoughts; and (v) the observation, that unresolved issues of the patient are re-enacted in the therapeutic setting, where they can be identified, discussed, interpreted, and modified.

The different types of psychodynamic psychotherapy reach from insight-oriented psychotherapy, which uncovers repressed, unconscious thoughts and feelings, and aims to enhance patient's autonomy, to supportive psychotherapy, which aims to suppress anxiety-provoking material and to foster ego functions and adaptive defenses (Lewin 2005). Supportive psychotherapy is more often indicated for patients in a palliative phase of their illness, as for most of these patients, the objective is to enhance adaptation, to diminish dysfunctional coping, to decrease psychological distress, and to restore psychological well-being (Guex et al. 2000; Rodin and Gillies 2000; Stiefel et al. 1998). Insight-oriented therapy is suitable for less vulnerable patients with intact ego functions, who are motivated to explore their thoughts and feelings in order to enhance reflection, and have the capacity to analyze adverse events (Rodin and Gillies 2000). A special form of psychodynamic psychotherapy is the Psychodynamic Life Narrative (PLN), which can be understood as a way to conceptualize maladaptive responses to physical illness. PLN aims to help the patient to understand their current psychological reactions to illness by linking it to important elements of their life trajectory (Viederman 1983; Viederman and Perry 1980). This type of therapy provides the patient with an opportunity to enhance a sense of control and coherence when facing illness (Viederman 2000).

With regard to the content of therapeutic interventions, the occurrence of cancer is not conceived as being the sole focus of the encounter with the patient, but other questions, such as how the specific reaction of the patient toward disease can be understood or why his relationships have been modified by the disease, are addressed (Krenz et al. 2013, submitted). A given psychological symptom is not just a target to suppress, since psychodynamic therapies aim to understand its underlying meaning: for example, it would be important for a psychodynamic-oriented therapist to understand whether the depressed mood of a women with breast cancer is due to the fact that she feels pressured by an increasing difficulty to fulfill her duties (loss of pre-existing capacities), to a modification of her self-image (loss of her breast), or to an alteration of her relationship with her husband (loss of commitment to the relationship). Depending on the source of the depressive symptoms, the therapeutic approach would be different, focusing on diminishing superego pressure, (pre-existing) difficulties with self-esteem or construction, and meaning of relationships.

While there are only few clinical trials evaluating the effectiveness of psychodynamic therapies in the physically ill (Ando et al. 2007, Ludwig et al. 2013, submitted), several single cases studies have been published over the past few years (Lacy and Higgings 2005; Redding 2005; Tepper et al. 2006).

3.3.2 Systemic Psychotherapy

Systemic psychotherapy is based on general systems theory, which conceives a system, such as the family, as organized and tries to understand the functions of its different elements, and their interrelations. Therefore, systemic psychotherapy views social coexistence of people as a complex and integrated whole, which is greater than the sum of its parts (Minuchin 1988; Sameroff 1983). Family therapists utilize special techniques and focus on variables, such as cohesion and hierarchy of the family, as well as attributed roles and implicit and explicit rules (Bressoud et al. 2007). Family members are considered to be helpful resources to by the patient, who can assist him in decision making and provide emotional and practical support (Xiaolian et al. 2002), but who may at times also be the source of conflict and suffering (Lyons et al. 1995).

In a report on the evidence of systemic family therapy, Stratton (2005) indicates that systemic therapy started with a common basis, but has over the past 50 years grown in various directions, with the most significant specific interventions belonging to the work of Bateson and the Palo Alto team (Jackson 1968a, b), the family structural therapy by Minuchin (1974), the strategic family therapy developed by Haley (1976) and Madanes (1981), and the approaches of Selvini Palazzoli and the Milan team (1978, 1991).

Being a systemic therapist does not imply that clinical care is restricted to social systems; systemic therapists also treat individual patients, but they are probably more sensitive to achieve an integrated systemic perspective in the analysis of the patient's problem and address more systematically intergenerational and intrafamilial problems and resources. Family response to illness is an important feature of systemic therapy with the physically ill: for example family myths—beliefs about a family member, such as «he has always been quickly irritated and prone to give up»—and family paradigms, such as «we function best by denying disagreements and avoiding difficulties», play an important role in systemic therapies.

Examples of scientifically evaluated systemic therapies in the medical and oncology setting are the Medical Family Therapy (Doherty et al. 1994) and the Family-Focused-Grief Therapy (FFGT), a preventive intervention for high-risk families (Kissane et al. 2006). FFGT is based on the assumption that the family is the primary provider of care for the terminally ill patient and that the type of functioning of the family is essential for the patient (Kissane et al. 1996a, b). Its aim is to optimize family functioning and to facilitate common grief. FFGT is a time-limited intervention (four to eight sessions of 90 min each), over a 9–18 month period, based on a manual with specific guidelines and clinical illustrations; its efficacy has been demonstrated in a randomized controlled trial (Kissane et al. 2006).

An other systemic approach, which has been examined in mostly qualitative research, is narrative therapy developed by Michael White and David Epston (White and Epston 1990). Narrative therapy is based on the concept that our identity is shaped by narratives and stories that we tell ourselves and others. Reality is thus a co-construction between different individuals, and the relational consensus produces the judgment that a perception is acceptable or not. Thus, not only the mind creates impressions based on observations, but confirmations of these impressions are sought with members of the society, the family or other systems, leading to interpersonal exchange which finally colors the way we perceive life. Therefore, the way a patient perceives his cancer, and the way he talks about it to his family or to medical professionals, will influence the perception and meaning he attributes to the disease and thus the psychological impact the situation will have. Narrative therapy implies that the patient is motivated to explicitly verbalize his thoughts and feelings with regard to the current situation, to communicate how he relates them to his life history and to evaluate the meaning he attributes to his disease in light of his trajectory.

In addition, systemic psychotherapy plays an important role in the treatment of childhood cancer, childhood cancer survivors, and their families. For example, Kazak (1989) found that multifamily group intervention reduced the posttraumatic stress symptoms and anxiety in childhood cancer survivors and their families. Furthermore Martire et al. (2004) demonstrated that systemic interventions for people with chronic illness (including cancer) were more effective than standard care».

3.3.3 Cognitive Behavioral Psychotherapy

Cognitive behavioral therapy (CBT) is a general term for several forms of therapies with similar characteristics, such as cognitive therapy, behavior therapy, rational emotive therapy, schema focused therapy, dialectical behavior therapy, mindfulness, motivational therapy, or cognitive–behavioral stress management. These interventions intend to reduce psychological distress and enhance adaptive coping by modifying maladaptive thoughts and behaviors, by raising awareness of emotional states and their connection with thoughts and behaviors, and by providing new skills (Hollon and Beck 2004).

CBT assumes that thoughts, behaviors, and emotions are at the base of human well-being and of the etiology and persistence of psychological disorders. For example, individual responses to illness are influenced by cognitive factors such as symptom perception (Lacroix et al. 1991), and variability in emotional reactions and self-care behaviors can be partly explained by disease-specific illness representations (Petrie et al. 1996; Prohaska et al. 1987). Or, the same situation encountered when feeling sad or happy will be followed by very different thoughts and behaviors (Segal et al. 2002). While it becomes more and more current in western healthcare to promote active self-management in patients (Tattersall 2002), CBT, which focuses on analysis of the function of the symptoms, skills acquisition, and increasing the autonomy of the patient, has been proposed as beneficial for patients with comorbid physical and psychological difficulties.

CBT offers several models for the somatic setting and patients with chronic medical problems. For example Acceptance and Commitment Therapy (ACT), an approach developed by Steven Hayes and colleagues (Hayes et al. 1999), is based on the concept that (i) instead of «controlling» our thoughts and feelings, we could choose to observe and accept them as they are and (ii) instead of putting our energy in avoiding our problems, we could act in the direction of personal values. For example, a patient with cancer might consider that if he is not cured, his life is meaningless, and he might avoid to be active due to fears of suffering from certain symptoms due to his cancer or its treatment: in ACT he would be invited to observe his emotions and thoughts inducing avoidance, and to reflect on the question whether «avoiding» is a strategy that really helps him in the long run. By investigating his values he might find reasons and motivation to confront life again, for example by connecting to other people, sharing his thoughts and emotions, or discovering new aspects of life.

CBT can be used as individual or group treatment and therapists feel free to follow a model, or to integrate different techniques (e.g., relaxation, exposure, meaning seeking) depending on the needs of the patient. As in other therapeutic approaches, the therapeutic relationship is an important part of CBT which is utilized by the therapist, for example by working on what happens in the therapeutic relationship and how this can be understood in light of the patient's difficulties.

CBT strives to be evidence based and much effort has been put in scientific research, including large randomized controlled studies. In patients suffering from cancer, CBT has been demonstrated to improve anxiety and depressive symptoms, self-esteem, immune functions, quality of life, optimism, self-efficacy, compliance, coping effectiveness and satisfaction, and to decrease cancer-related fatigue, cortisol levels, pain, and distress (Andersen et al. 2007; Daniels and Kissane 2008; Greer et al. 1992; Hopko et al. 2005; Lee et al. 2006; Manne et al. 2007; Mefford et al. 2007; Moorey et al. 1998; Osborn et al. 2006; Penedo et al. 2007; Tatrow 2006; Witek-Janusek et al. 2008; Wojtyna et al. 2007).

3.3.4 Psychotherapy Integration

The first official comment on the need to integrate different psychotherapeutic approaches to best serve patients could be attributed to Freud when he stated that psychoanalytic technique alone seems insufficient for certain patients: «these patients cannot bring out the material necessary for resolving their phobia so long as they feel protected by obeying the condition which it lays down», only after they learned to no longer need the protection of their phobia, «does the material become accessible, which, when it has been mastered, leads to a solution of the phobia» (Freud 1910/1975, p 145). This comment can be understood as showing that Freud realized that, for some patients, psychoanalytic interpretation alone might not be enough and that an alternative approach might be necessary before interpretation (Trijsburg et al. 2005). Nowadays, neither monism (psychotherapeutic modalities have unique qualities differentiating them) or specificity (one intervention has one intended result), nor eclecticism (interventions are effective irrespective of the particular theory from which they derive) or universality (common factors among psychotherapeutic treatments) can adequately reflect clinical reality in its totality, instead it is considered that specific interventions reinforce common factors, and common factors reinforce the effects of specific interventions (Strupp and Hadley 1979).

Integrative approaches are more and more practiced, with one-half to two-thirds of clinicians working with a variety of concepts derived from several theoretical schools (Lambert et al. 2004). A survey, conducted in the Netherlands with 1143 therapists from various orientations found that self-declared monotherapists of all orientations use interventions from other theoretical approaches (Trijsburg et al. 2004).

Four ways to integrate psychotherapies have been identified: (i) technical eclecticism, which uses the combination of different interventions without adopting the underlying theoretical models, (ii) theoretical integration, which synthesizes existing theories in a new structure with its own theoretical framework, (iii) common factors approach, which combines core elements that are common to all psychotherapies, and (iv) assimilative integration, grounded in one psychotherapeutic approach, but integrating practices from other approaches (Norcross and Goldfried 2005). Examples of common factors based on different studies (Grencavage and Norcross 1990; Lambert et al. 1994; Trijsburg et al. 2004) include therapist empathy, congruence, acceptance and involvement, patient expectations, hope, quality of communication, working alliance and engagement.

Several integrative psychotherapeutic approaches have been developed (e.g., the Common Factor Model of Arkowitz 1992; Interpersonal Therapy by Klerman et al. 1984; Cognitive analytic therapy by Ryle and Kerr 2002; Systematic Eclectic psychotherapy by Beutler and Consoli 1992; Multimodal therapy by Lazarus 1989, 2005; Kissane's cognitive-existential group therapy 1997). Psycho-oncology could benefit from this work, for which encouraging results have been found endorsing the common factors theory in cancer care and the effectiveness of technical eclecticism and theoretical integration (Liossi and White 2001; McLean et al. 2013; Schnur and Montgomery 2010).

4   Outcome of Psycho-Oncological Interventions

Outcome of psycho-oncological interventions are not easy to determine, since some patients value a decrease of distressing symptoms, such as feelings of depressed mood, while others emphasize personal growth, finding meaning in a situation perceived as chaotic, or improved interpersonal relationships and communication. Up to now, most studies evaluate outcome with traditional psychometric assessments, which do not necessarily reflect the therapeutic process and might not be relevant to all psychotherapeutic approaches, such as the psychodynamic approach (Krenz et al. 2013, submitted).

While there is a real need for creativity with regard to the evaluation of individual psycho-oncological interventions, outcomes for partners and family members have also been neglected.

Finally psycho-oncological interventions seem to influence treatment adherence, but its relevance for survival is controversial (Chow et al. 2004; Smedslund and Ringdal 2004; Spiegel et al. 1989). A systematic Cochrane review examining the effectiveness of psychosocial interventions in breast cancer patients on survival outcome showed insufficient evidence for such an effect (Edwards et al. 2008). Possible pathways for prolonging survival, taking into account adherence to treatment, self-care, or enhanced immune system, might deserve attention. For example, it is known that mood disturbance is associated with poorer response to chemotherapy (Walker et al. 1999), and that feelings of helplessness or hopelessness are associated with poorer survival (Watson et al. 1999).

5   Conclusions

For different psycho-oncological and psychotherapeutic interventions, clinical validity and scientific evidence have been demonstrated. Since existing psychological interventions which have been proven to be beneficial can easily be adapted to cancer patients, it seems that instead of conceiving new interventions for the oncology setting, and thus reinvent the wheel, it is more relevant to identify patients who benefit from specific psycho-oncological interventions and to develop and implement programs that cover the spectrum of treatment modalities, which can than be evaluated with regard to effectiveness (Ludwig et al. 2013, submitted).

References

Andersen BL, Farrar WB, Golden-Kreutz D et al (2007) Distress reduction from a psychological intervention contributes to improved health for cancer patients. Brain Behav Immun 21(7):953–961

Ando M, Tsuda A, Morita T (2007) Life review interview on the spiritual well-being of terminally ill cancer patients. Support Care Cancer 15:225–231

Arkowitz H (1992) A common factors therapy for depression. In: Norcorss JC, Goldfried MR (eds) Handbook of psychotherapy integration. Basic Books, New York, pp 402–432

Beutler LE, Consoli AJ (1992) Integration through fundamental similarities and useful differences among schools. In: Norcross JC, Goldfried MR (eds) Handbook of psychotherapy integration. Basic Books, New York, pp 202–231

Bressoud A, Real del Sarte O, Stiefel F et al (2007) Impact of family structure on long-term survivors of osteosarcoma. Support Care Cancer 15:525–531

Chow E, Tsao MN, Harth T (2004) Does psychosocial intervention improve survival in cancer? A meta-analysis. Palliat Med 18:25–31

Daniels J, Kissane DW (2008) Psychosocial interventions for cancer patients. Curr Opin Oncol 20:367–371

Devine EC, Westlake SK (1995) The effects of psychoeducational care provided to adults with cancer: meta-analysis of 116 studies. Oncol Nurs Forum 22:1369–1381

Doherty WJ, McDaniel SH, Hepworth J (1994) Medical family therapy: an emerging arena for family therapy. J Fam Ther 16:31–46

Edwards AGK, Hubert-Williams N, Neal RD (2008) Psychological interventions for women with metastatic breast cancer (Review). Cochrane database of systematic reviews 3

Faulkner A, Maguire P (1994) Talking to cancer patients and their relatives. Oxford University Press, New York

Franck JD, Frank JB (1991) Persuasion and healing: a comparative study of psychotherapy. John Hopkins Universtiy Press, Baltimore

Frank J (1988) What is Psychotherapy? In: Bloch S (ed) An Introduction to the Psychotherapies. Oxford University Press, Oxford [1979]

Freud S (1910/1975) The future prospects of psycho-analytic therapy. In: Strachey J (ed and trans) The standard edition of the complete psychological works of Sigmund Freud, vol 11. Oxford University Press, Oxford, pp 139–151

Greer S, Moorey S, Baruch JD et al (1992) Adjuvant psychological therapy for patients with cancer: a prospective randomised trial. Br Med J 304:675–680

Grencavage LM, Norcross JC (1990) Where are the communalities among therapeutic common factors? Prof Psychol Res Pract 21:278–372

Guex P, Stiefel F, Rousselle I (2000) Psychotherapy for the patient with cancer. Psychother rev 2:269–273

Haley J (1976) Problem-solving therapy: new strategies for effective family therapy. Josey Bass, San Francisco

Hayes SC, Strosahl KD, Wilson KG (1999) Acceptance and commitment therapy: an experiential approach to behavior change. The Guilford Press, NewYork

Hellbom M, Brandberg Y, Glimelius B et al (1998) Individual psychological support for cancer patients: utilisation and patient satisfaction. Patient Educ Couns 34:247–256

Hollon SD, Beck AT (2004) Cognitive and cognitive behavioral therapies. In: Lambert MJ (ed) Bergin and Garfied's handbook of psychotherapy and behavior change, 5th edn. Wiley, New York

Hopko DR, Bell JL, Armento MEA et al (2005) Behavior therapy for depressed cancer patients in primary care. Psychother Theory Res Pract Train 42:236–243

Jackson DD (1968a) Human communication, T.1: communication, family and marriage. Science and Behavior Books, Palo Alto

Jackson DD (1968b) Human communciation,T.2: communcation, family and marriage. Science and Behavior Books, Palo Alto

Kaplan HI, Sadock BJ (1998) Kaplan and Sadock's synopsis of psychiatry: behavioral sciense/ clinical psychitary, 8th edn. Williams and Wilkins, Baltimore

Kazak AE (1989) Families of chronically ill children: a systems and social-ecological model of adaptation and challenge. J Consultation Clin Psychol 57:25–30

Kerrihard T, Breitbart W, Dent R et al (1999) Anxiety in patients with cancer and human inmmunodeficiency virus. Semin Clin Neuropsychiatry 4:114–132

Kissane DW, Bloch S, Dowe DL et al (1996a) The Melbourne family grief study, I: perceptions of family functioning in bereavement. Am J Psychiatry 153:650–658

Kissane DW, Bloch S, Dowe DL et al (1996b) The Melbourne family grief study, II: psychosocial morbidity and grief in bereaved families. Am J Psychiatry 153:659–666

Kissane DW, Bloch S, Miach P et al (1997) Cognitive-existential group therapy for patients with primary breast cancer–techniques and themes. Psychooncology 6:25–33

Kissane DW, Grabsch B, Love A et al (2004a) Psychiatric disorder in women with early stage and advanced breast cancer: a comparative analysis. Aust N Z J Psychiatry 38:320–326

Kissane DW, McKenzie M, Bloch S et al (2006) Family focused grief therapy: a randomized, controlled trial in palliative care and bereavement. Am J Psychiatry 163:1208–1218

Kissane DW, Wein S, Love A et al (2004b) The demoralization scale. A report of its development and preliminary validation. J Palliat Care 20:269–276

Klerman G, Weissman M, Rousevill B et al (1984) Interpersonal psychotherapy of depression. Basic Books, New York

Krenz S, Sodel C, Stagno A et al. (2013) Psychodynamic interventions in cancer care II: a qualitative analysis of the therapists' reports (submitted)

Lacroix JM, Martin B, Avendano M et al (1991) Symptom schemata in chronic respiratory patients. Health Psychol 10:268–273

Lacy TJ, Higgins MJ (2005) Integrated medical-psychiatric care of a dying patient: a case of dynamically informed 'practical psychotherapy'. J Am Acad Psychoanal Dyn Psychiatry 33:619–636

Lambert MJ, Bergin AE (1994) The effectiveness of psychotherpy. In: Bergin AE, Garfield SL (eds) Handbook of psychotherapy and behavoir change, 4th edn. New York, Wiley, pp 143–189

Lambert MJ, Ogles BM (2004) The efficacy and effectiveness of psychotherapy. In: Lambert MJ (ed) Bergin and Garfield's handbook of psychotherapy and behavior change, 5th edn. Wiley, New York

Lambert MJ, Bergin AE, Garfield SL (2004) Introduction and historical overview. In: Lambert MJ (ed) Bergin and Garfield's handbook of psychotherapy and behavior change, 5th edn. New York, Wiley, pp 3–15

Lazarus AA (1989) The practice of multimodal therapy. Systematic, comprehensive, and effective psychotherapy. Johns Hopkins University Press, Baltimore

Lazarus AA (2005) Multimodal therapy. In: Norcross JC, Goldfried MR (eds) Handbook of psychotherapy integration, 2nd edn. New York, Oxford, pp 105–120

Lee V, Cohen SR, Edgar L et al (2006) Meaning—making intervention during breast or colorectal cancer treatment improves self-esteem, optimism, and self-efficacy. Soc Sci Med 62:3133–3145

Lewin K (2005) The theoretical basis of dynamic psychiatry. In: Gabbard GO (ed) Psychodynamic psychiatry in clinical practice: the DSM-IV edition. American Psychiatric Press, Washington

Liossi C, White P (2001) Efficacy of clinical hypnosis in the enhancement of quality of life of terminally ill cancer patients. Contemp Hypn 18:145–160

Ludwig S, Krenz S, Zdrojewski C et al (2013) Psychodynamic interventions in cancer care I: psychometric results of a randomized controlled trial (submitted)

Lyons RF, Sullivan MJL, Ritvo PG (1995) Relationships in chronic illness and disability. Sage Publications, Thousand Oaks

Madanes C (1981) Strategic family therapy. Josey Bass, San Francisco

Manne SL, Rubin S, Edelson M et al (2007) Coping and communication-enhancing intervention versus supportive counseling for women diagnosed with gynecologic cancers. J Consult Clin Psychol 75:615–628

Martire L, Lustig A, Schultz R et al (2004) Is it beneficial to involve a family member? A meta-analysis of psychosocial interventions for chronic illness. Health Psychol 23:599–611

Massie MJ (2004) Prevalence of depression in patients with cancer. J Natl Cancer Inst Monogr 32:57–71. doi:10.1093/jncimonographs/lgh014

McLean LM, Walton T, Rodin G et al (2013) A couple-based intervention for patients and caregivers facing end-stage cancer: outcomes of a randomized controlled trial. Psychooncology 22:28–38

Mefford K, Nichols JF, Pakiz B et al (2007) A cognitive behavioral therapy intervention to promote weight loss improves body composition and blood lipid profiles among overweight breast cancer survivors. Breast Cancer Res Treat 104:145–152

Meyer TJ, Mark MM (1995) Effects of psychosocial interventions with adult cancer patients: a meta-analysis of randomized experiments. Health Psychol 14:101–108

Minuchin P (1988) Relationships within the family: a systems perspective on development. In: Hinde RA, Stevenson-Hinde J (eds) Relationships within families: mutual influences. Wiley, New York

Minuchin S (1974) Families and famliy therapy. Harvard university, Cambridge

Mitchell AJ, Chan M, Bhatti H et al (2011) Prevalence of depression, anxiety, and adjustment disorder in oncological, heamatological, and palliative-care settings: a meta-analysis of 94 interview-based studies. Lancet Oncol 12:160–174

Moorey S, Greer S, Bliss J et al (1998) A comparison of adjuvant psychological therapy and supportive sounselling in patients with cancer. Psychooncology 7:218–228

Norcross JC, Goldfried MR (eds) (2005) Handbook of psychotherapy integration, 2nd edn. Oxford, New York

Osborn RL, Demoncada AC, Feurerstein M (2006) Psychosocial interventions for depression, anxiety, and quality of life in cancer survivors: meta-analyses. Int J Psychiatry Med 36:13–34

Penedo FJ, Traeger L, Dahn J et al (2007) Cognitive behavioral stress management intervention improves quality of life in Spanish monolingual Hispanic men treated for localized prostate cancer: results of a randomized controlled trial. Int J Behav Med 12:164–172

Petrie KJ, Weinman J, Sharpe N et al (1996) Roles of patients' view of their illness in predicting return to work and functioning after myocardial infarction: longitudinal study. Br Med J 312:1191–1194

Pirl WF (2004) Evidence report on the occurrence, assessement, and treatment of depression in cancer patients. J Natl Cancer Inst Monogr 32:32–39. doi:10.1093/jncimonographs/lgh026

Prohaska TR, Keller ML, Leventhal EA et al (1987) Impact of symptoms and aging attribution on emotions and coping. Health Psychol 6:495–514

Razavi D, Stiefel F (1994) Common psychiatric disorders in cancer patients. I. Adjustment disorders and depressive disorders. J Support Care Cancer 2:223–232

Redding KK (2005) When death becomes the end of an analytic treatment. Clin Work Soc J 33:69–79

Rodin G, Gillies LA (2000) Individual psychotherapy for the patient with advanced disease. In: Ghochinov HM, Breitbart WGO (eds) Handbook of psychiatry in palliative medicine. Oxford University Press, New York

Ryle A, Kerr I (2002) Introducing cognitive analytic therapy: principles and practice. Wiley, Chichester

Sameroff AJ (1983) Developmental systems: context and evolution. In: Mussen PH, Kessen W (ed) Handbook of child psychology: history, theory, and methods, 4th edn. Wiley, New York

Schnur JB, Montgomery GH (2010) A systematic review of therapeutic alliance, group cohesion, empathy, and goal consensus/collaboration in psychotherapeutic interventions in cancer: uncommon factors? Clin Psychol Rev 30:238–247

Segal Z, Teasdale J, Williams M (2002) Mindfulness-based cognitive therapy for depression. Guilford Press, New York

Selvini Palazzoli M (1978) Self starvation: from the individual to family therapy. Aronson, New York

Selvini Palazzoli M (1991) Team consultation: an indispensable tool for the process of knowledge. J Fam Ther 13:31–53

Sheard T, Maguire P (1999) The effect of psychological interventions on anxiety and depression in cancer patients: results of two meta-analyses. Br J Cancer 80:1770–1780

Smedslunc G, Ringdal GI (2004) Meta-analysis of the effects of psychosocial interventions on survival time in cancer patients. J Psychosom Res 57:123–131

Spiegel D, Bloom JR, Kraemer HC et al (1989) Effect of psychosocial treatment on survival of patients with metastatic breast cancer. Lancet 2:888–891

Stiefel F, Guex P, Real O (1998) An introduction to psycho-oncology with special emphasis to its historical and cultural context. In: Bruera E, Portenoy R (eds) Topics in palliative care 3. Oxford University Press, New York

Stratton P (2005) Report on the evidence base of systemic family therapy. Association for family therapy

Strupp HH, Hadley SW (1979) Specific vs. Nonspecific factors in psychotherapy. Arch Gen Psychiatry 36:1125–1136

Tatrow K, Montgomery GH (2006) Cognitive behavioral therapy for distress and pain in breast cancer patients: a meta-analysis. J Behav Med 29:17–27

Tattersall RL (2002) The expert patient: a new approach to chronic disease management for the twenty-first century. Clin Med 2:227–229

Tepper MC, Dodes LM, Wool CA et al (2006) A psychotherapy dominated by separation, termination, and death. Harv Rev Psychiatry 14:257–267

Trijsburg RW, Colijn S, Holmes J (2005) Psychotherapy integration. In: Gabbard GO, Beck JS, Holmes J (ed) Oxford textbook of psychotherapy. Oxford, New York

Trijsburg RW, Lietaer G, Colijn S et al (2004) Construct validity of the comprehensive psychotherapeutic interventions rating scale. Psychother Res 14:346–366

Viederman M (1983) The psychodynamic life narrative: a psychotherapeutic intervention useful in crisis situations. Psychiatry 46:236–246

Viederman M (2000) The supportive relationship, the psychodynamic life narrative, and the dying patient. In: Chochinov HM, Breitbart WGO (eds) Handbook of psychiatry in palliative medicine. Oxford University Press, New York

Viederman M, Perry SW (1980) Use of a psychodynamic life narrative in the treatment of depression in the physically ill. Gen Hosp Psychiatry 2:177–185

Walker LG, Walker MB, Ogston K et al (1999) Psychological, clinical and pathological effects of relaxation training and guided imagery during primary chemotherapy. Br J Cancer 80:262–268

Wampold BE (2001) The great psychotherapy debate: models, methods and findings. Mahwah NJ, Lawrence erlbaum associates

Watson M, Haviland JS, Greer S et al (1999) Influence of psychological response on survival in breast cancer: a population-based cohort sutdy. Lancet 354:1331–1336

White M, Epston D (1990) Narrative means to therapeutic ends. WW Norton, New York

Witek-Janusek L, Albuquerque K, Chroniak KR et al (2008) Effect of mindfulness based stress reduction on immune function, quality of life and coping in women newly diagnosed with early stage breast cancer. Brain Behav Immun 22:969–981

Wojtyna E, Zycinska J, Stawiarska P (2007) The influence of cognitive-behaviour therapy on quality of life and self-esteem in women suffering from breast cancer. Rep Pract Oncol Radiother 12:109–117

Xiaolian J, Chaiwan S, Panuthai S et al (2002) Family support and self-care behaviour of Chinese chronic obstructive pulmonary disease patients. Nurs Health Sci 4:41–49

Zabora J, Brintzenhogeszoc K, Love A et al (2001) The prevalence of psychosocial distress by cancer site. Psychooncology 10:19–28

Quality of Life in Oncology

Ute Goerling and Anna Stickel

Abstract

Continuous improvements in the diagnosis and treatment of cancer lead to improved cure rates and longer survival. However, in many patients, the disease becomes chronic. In this context, the patients' quality of life (QOL) becomes a crucial issue. After an introduction about QOL, results from different areas of cancer treatment are presented considering their impact on QOL. Finally, implications are discussed for researchers, clinicians, and patients.

U. Goerling (✉) · A. Stickel
Department of Psychooncology, Charité Comprehensive Cancer Center, Berlin, Germany
e-mail: ute.goerling@charite.de

A. Stickel
e-mail: anna.stickel@charite.de

U. Goerling (ed.), *Psycho-Oncology*, Recent Results in Cancer Research 197,   137
DOI: 10.1007/978-3-642-40187-9_10, © Springer-Verlag Berlin Heidelberg 2014

Contents

1   Introduction.. 138
2   What Exactly is Quality of Life? 138
    2.1   Terms and Definitions... 138
    2.2   Measures in Quality of Life.. 139
3   Quality of Life During Oncological Treatment 142
    3.1   Surgery.. 142
    3.2   Chemotherapy 143
    3.3   Radiotherapy 143
4   Relevance of Quality of life 144
    4.1   Relevance for Researchers.. 144
    4.2   Implications for Clinicians.. 145
    4.3   Significance for People Affected by Cancer................................... 146
5   Challenges in Quality of Life-Measurements 147
6   Quality of Life of Health Care Providers 148
7   Summary.. 149
References.. 149

> *Sittin' on the front porch*
> *ice cream in my hand*
> *meltin' in the sun*
> *all that chocolate on my tongue*
> *and that's good enough reason to live*
> *good enough reason to live....*
> *And if I die young, at least I got some chocolate on my tongue...*
> *(The Wood Brothers 2006).*

1   Introduction

Quality of life (QOL)—everyone knows what it is, but it probably means something different to each individual. For some, being able to travel to foreign countries is important for their appraisal of good QOL, for others, it is having time for their hobbies or enjoying little things like the pleasure of chocolate melting on one's tongue.

In the face of a chronic disease QOL is an issue of special value. Cancer and its treatment are debilitating and thus have an impact on QOL, depending on the individual's perception of the situation. Cancer care has become more successful, yet also more complicated. Therefore, understanding what cancer survival means to patients is an important intention in current research (see also "Cancer survivorship in adults"). Not only the efficacy of treatments but also their toxicity and associated problems for the patients are receiving increasing attention.

Many parameters elucidating the effects of cancer are not quantifiable with laboratory tests or imaging procedures. Therefore, variables such as social functioning, sense of well-being, fatigue, or global QOL are ascertained by self-reports. These self-reports add to the picture of biomedical outcomes and are important for gaining a better understanding of the consequences of cancer and its treatments (Osoba 2011).

Thus apart from objective criteria like survival time, time to recurrence, side effects, etc., the interest in patients' experiences has grown and their subjective perceptions of living with cancer are valued more.

2   What Exactly is Quality of Life?

2.1   Terms and Definitions

Different terms and definitions revolve around the rather elusive multidimensional construct: Patient function, health status, life satisfaction, QOL, health-related quality of life (HRQOL), or patient-reported outcomes. Yet there is no universal definition (Leplège and Hunt 1997).

QOL is always highly individual. It depends on the present lifestyle, past experiences, future hopes, dreams, and ambitions. QOL should include all aspects of life and experiences in life and take account of disease and treatment. An individual has a good QOL, when experiences are in accordance to hopes. The opposite is true when the experiences of the individual makes do not match the hopes that he/she cherishes. QOL is time-dependent and gives information about the difference between hopes or expectations of the individual and his/her experiences at a given moment (Calmann 1984).

Already Aristotle (384–322 BC) refers to the fundamental problem of QOL-research: "and often the same person changes his mind: when he becomes ill, it is health, and as long as he is healthy it is money". Patients may change their personal scale about what is important in the course of their disease and the question is how?

In 1993 the World Health Organization published the following definition:

> Quality of life is defined as an individual's perception of their position in life in the context of the culture and value systems in which they live and in relation to their goals, expectations, standards and concerns. It is a broad ranging concept affected in a complex way by the person's physical health, psychological state, level of independence, social relationships, and their relationship to salient features of their environment. (WHO 1993, p 153).

To distinguish QOL of the general population from the QOL of patients the term "HRQOL" was introduced. A more inclusive term however is "patient reported outcomes" which comprises any feedback given directly by the patient, e.g., satisfaction with care (Osoba 2011).

2.2   Measures in Quality of Life

A proper estimation of QOL is challenging. Already 100 years ago there were efforts to include aspects of QOL in the use and evaluation of medical treatment.

"Health is a state of complete physical, mental, and social well-being and not merely the absence of disease or infirmity" (WHO 1946).

Early evaluation instruments of QOL focused on physical aspects of disease (Fayers and Bottomley 2002). In 1948, the American oncologist David A. Karnofsky developed an index that allows the doctor to give an estimation of the patient's physical condition on a scale (Karnofsky index, Karnofsky and Burchenal 1949). Another observer-rated assessment of QOL in oncology was developed by Spitzer. The doctor can value the activity, daily life, health, social support, and future perspective of the patient and create a total score. However, this time economic method has a significant drawback: it is open to different interpretations (Spitzer et al. 1981). Later the patients' expectations, perceptions as well as values received increasing attention and emotional and social aspects were added in assessments (Schumacher et al. 1991)

Today, self-reports are considered more appropriate than observer ratings of QOL. The questionnaires need to be short but nevertheless sensitive. They should allow cross-disease comparisons but also assess the specific nature of a certain disease. Finally, they must be reliable and valid.

Since 1964 certain projects in the United States assessing the needs and QOL of healthy individuals aim at resolving long-term deficits. The National Cancer Institute confirms that all clinical trials should include QOL as an outcome measure since 1991.

In the endeavor to improve QOL-research, several institutions created groups to give advice on the design, implementation, and analysis of QOL studies. For example the Quality of Life Group (QLG) of the European Organization for Research and Treatment of Cancer (EORTC) was established in 1980 (Fayers and Bottomley 2002). One of the group's main achievements is the development and continual improvement of the QOL Questionnaire. Its brief core measure includes a global health status/QOL scale, functional scales, symptom scales, and several single questions on frequently reported symptoms, and financial concerns (see Table 1).

The 30-item core instrument should be supplemented by modules specific to a tumor site, treatment modality, or additional QOL dimensions. The modules which have already been validated are presented in Table 2. The QLQ-C30 and QLQ modules are applicable cross-culturally as they are available in many different languages and are the most extensively used questionnaires in clinical trials in Europe (Fayers and Bottomley 2002).

In North America, the predominantly used tool is the Functional Assessment of Cancer Therapy Scale. Its general version (FACT-G, Version 3) has 27 items from which the subscales physical, social, emotional, and functional well-being can be derived (Cella et al. 2002; Cella et al. 1993) and which can be summed to a total score. Additionally, a broad range of tumor-, treatment-, or symptom-specific modules can be used (Luckett et al. 2011).

These two most widely used tools differ in scale structure, social domains, and tone. Their psychometric properties are comparable and thus cannot be used as a criterion in selecting one of these questionnaires (Luckett and King 2010).

Table 1 The EORTC core questionnaire

		Number of Items
QLQ-C30	Global health status	2
	Functional Scales	
	Physical functioning	5
	Role functioning	2
	Emotional functioning	4
	Social functioning	2
	Cognitive functioning	2
	Symptom Scales	
	Fatigue	3
	Nausea and vomiting	2
	Pain	2
	Dyspnoea	1
	Insomnia	1
	Appetite loss	1
	Constipation	1
	Diarrhea	1
	Financial impact	1

Furthermore, item banks and computerized adaptive testing (CAT) have been developed to gain a more comprehensive coverage of QOL issues (Cella et al. 2007). The Patient-Reported Outcomes Measurement Information System (PROMIS) was funded by the National Institutes of Health (NIH) and aims to enable an efficient, flexible, and precise measurement of PROs (http://www.nihpromis.org/).

3 Quality of Life During Oncological Treatment

Treatments differ in their impact on QOL. In the case of various treatment options with curative objective, relapse free survival was previously considered as the only target criterion. Again, QOL must be seen as an important parameter and should be discussed with the patient. Efforts in early diagnosis, state-of-the-art diagnostics, and multimodal therapy concepts prolong survival time, but what is the price the patient has to pay? Which of the therapies offering an improved life expectancy is superior considering their impact on QOL? Is a treatment, which is less effective but also less detrimental to QOL more preferable than an aggressive therapy? The same thoughts apply to palliative treatment options. How much QOL does a person need to endure survival 8 weeks longer?

Table 2 The EORTC modules

Modules (validated)	Name*
Bone metastases	QLQ-BM 22
Brain cancer	QLQ-BN 20
Cervical cancer	QLQ-CX 24
Colorectal cancer	QLQ-CR 29
Colorectal liver metastases	QLQ-LMC 21
Endometrial	QLQ-EN 24
Gastric cancer	QLQ-STO 22
Head and neck	QLQ-H&N 35
Hepatocellular carcinoma	QLQ-HCC 18
Information	QLQ-INFO 25
Lung	QLQ-LC 13
Multiple myeloma	QLQ-MY 20
Neuroendocrine carcinoid	QLQ-GINET 21
Esophageal cancer	QLQ-OES 18
Esophageal-gastric cancer	QLQ-OG 25
Ovarian	QLQ-OV 28
Prostate	QLQ-PR 25

*The number after the abbreviation indicates the number of items

Thus the selection of tools for assessing QOL should also be determined by the treatment choice. For example one questionnaire was developed specifically for patients after high dose chemotherapy in palliative care (Sprangers et al. 1998) or a module was created to detect cancer-related fatigue, which can occur as a side effect but also as a long-term consequence of the antitumor therapy (Weis et al. 2013).

Below we will briefly discuss QOL-research in selected areas of oncologic therapy. This—by no means exhaustive—overview aims to demonstrate the complexity, diversity, and problems of QOL issues.

3.1 Surgery

The influence of surgical approaches on QOL has been examined in the context of different tumor entities. Interventions changing the body image are of particular interest. A number of studies for example examine the impact the creation of an anus praeter has on QOL (Grumann et al. 2001; Mrak et al. 2011). For almost 100 years the abdominoperineal extirpation represented the standard therapy in surgery of rectal cancer (Pachler and Wille-Jorgensen 2012). In the context of the development and improvement of surgical techniques, and depending on the location of the tumor, an anterior sphincter-preserving resection then became the preferred treatment. This decision was not least due to the assumption that QOL is significantly better for patients whose sphincter function is preserved. In a systematic review on this topic, Pachler and Wille-Jorgensen (2012) evaluated 35 studies, matching their inclusion criteria, involving 5127 patients. None of the selected studies were randomized, 20 were retrospective and 15 prospective. Disease-specific instruments (e.g., EORTC-C30 and QLQ-C38, FACTC) were used in 23 studies. Seven studies used general questionnaires and five combined general with disease-specific questionnaires. Contrary to general expectations a total of 14 studies showed that patients after abdominoperineal extirpation do not have poorer QOL compared to patients after an anterior resection. A small influence due to a stoma could be found in three trials. In 12 studies patients who experienced an abdominoperineal extirpation showed a significantly poorer QOL on one or more subscales. However, in five studies a significantly better QOL was found in some subscales after anterior resection. One study describes an improved QOL in patients after abdominoperineal extirpation.

Comparisons of open versus laparoscopic surgery and robot-assisted surgery are further topics in literature (Bertani et al. 2011). King et al. (2006) compared the laparoscopic resection with the open resection of colorectal cancer in a randomized trial and came to the conclusion that patients have a shorter residence time in the hospital after laparoscopic resection. However, the groups did not differ concerning QOL.

A recent review on the outcome of oncoplastic breast-conserving surgery evaluated 88 studies (Haloua et al. 2013). Only one trial used QOL as an outcome measure (Veiga et al. 2010). This study compared the results of oncoplastic breast-conserving surgery with breast-conserving surgery, and concluded that oncoplastic surgery has a positive impact on QOL of women with breast cancer.

Little to no attention seems to be given to studies on the impact of palliative surgery on QOL.

3.2   Chemotherapy

Studies on QOL during chemotherapy with curative objective address nausea, vomiting, and fatigue, among other aspects. The negative impact of chemotherapy-induced nausea and vomiting despite antiemetic therapy could be shown in a multicenter study in various tumor entities (Fernández-Ortega et al. 2012). Chemotherapy in women with breast cancer was found to have a negative impact on cognition and fatigue (de Ruiter et al. 2011). The latter showed a poorer QOL compared to the patients with no indication for adjuvant chemotherapy. A further study comparing younger versus older adults with acute myeloid leukemia receiving an intensive chemotherapy showed a diminished QOL and physical function. However, the patients' age had no influence on QOL (Mohamedali et al. 2012).

Several studies can be found in the literature on the effect of therapy on QOL in systemic cancers in childhood, enabling an extended follow-up period (Kanellopoulos et al. 2013).

Drug trials often explore QOL in various treatment arms. Thus, given the same overall survival rate in different arms, treatment decisions can be made according to the results of QOL assessments. The question of using chemotherapy in palliative situations is especially challenging. Studies have demonstrated the willingness of patients to accept side effects while gaining relief from disease associated symptoms (Archer et al. 1999).

3.3   Radiotherapy

Radiotherapy is a further essential element in cancer treatment in curative, as well as palliative care, however, once again not without consequences for the patients' QOL. Fatigue is one of the most common side effects and late sequelae of radiotherapy. Research indicates that up to 80 % of the patients suffer from fatigue during and after radiotherapy (Jereczek-Fossa et al. 2002).

Due to the fact, that radiotherapy often is organ-preserving, the maintenance of a good QOL is expected. However, prospective studies on this subject are still rare. A review on the use of intensity-modulated radiotherapy in patients with head and neck cancer was able to detect only 10 studies in which QOL data was collected, out of 65 studies matching the search criteria (Scott-Brown et al. 2010). Only one study was randomized. According to its results, the expected positive impact of intensity-modulated radiotherapy versus conventional radiotherapy could not be detected. The authors assume that there is no relationship between loss of function and global QOL.

A further study with over 500 patients with head and neck cancer demonstrated that a quarter of patients treated with radiotherapy had more than 10 % weight loss, which was associated with a diminished QOL (Langius et al. 2013).

4   Relevance of Quality of life

4.1   Relevance for Researchers

"...oncology has generated some of the most productive research in medicine for the development and utilization of QoL measures." (Fallowfield 2009, p 2).

Although some clinical trials still do not discuss QOL issues, they have gained increasing attention in recent years. The methodology in HRQOL-research has improved and the compliance with its measurement has grown (Bottomley et al. 2005; Efficace et al. 2003). Several reviews about QOL studies examine their reporting standard, presentation, and interpretation for QOL (Bottomley et al. 2005; Brundage et al. 2011; Cocks et al. 2008) and different researchers have proposed guidelines for developing and evaluating study protocols (Cocks et al. 2011; Efficace et al. 2003)

The presentation of results in QOL-research has increasingly become a matter of debate as the meaningfulness of statistical significance has been questioned in the clinical context. Statistical significance cannot be equated with clinical significance, especially if the later was not defined a priori and used to determine the sample size for a trail (Cocks et al. 2008). Different guidelines have been published on how to rate the importance of change (Cocks et al. 2012; King 1996; King 2001; Osoba et al. 1998). It has been proposed that a change of 10 points on a scale from 0 to 100 (Osoba et al. 2005) or the 0.5 standard deviation (Norman et al. 2003) is clinically meaningful. However, the clinical interpretation of QOL differences is lacking as clinical significance is mostly not addressed in papers (Cocks et al. 2008).

A further problem is that QOL results are often published in separate papers. However, self-reports should complement standard biological endpoints (like tumor regression, time to progression, survival) and be described in a single publication (Osoba 2011).

Conflicting findings in comparative analyses of research results make unequivocal treatment decisions difficult for clinicians. Divergent results may occur through the use of different questionnaires. Hence a generic questionnaire may not be sensitive to differences, for example, in certain surgical procedures. Many studies lack the pretherapeutic assessment of QOL. Furthermore the influence of important factors such as social status, and gender differences remain unconsidered. In order to give careful consideration to these aspects, prospective, methodologically well-planned, and comprehensive studies are needed.

But how can we interpret results of QOL-research? Why does a patient with a colostomy rate his QOL as good as or better as a patient, whose natural anus could be preserved? Why does a woman after mastectomy evaluate her QOL as comparably good as a woman after breast-conserving surgery? These issues are known as the paradox of QOL-research in literature (Herschbach 2002).

As described above various dimensions are assessed in QOL-research. However, the patient's preference is often ignored, i.e., which dimensions are given more weight by which patient. Their ratings can vary considerably (Osoba 1994). Furthermore, the weighting of the dimensions may change over time. Ultimately the patient's expectations to the outcome of cancer therapy play a significant role, which arise from the comparison of the actual state and the desired state.

4.2 Implications for Clinicians

It has been criticized that study results are not receiving enough attention from clinicians and the routine assessment of QOL has not been implemented into clinical practice. There are fears that this might be too expensive or time-consuming. However, research has shown that the regular use of QOL measurements increases the practitioner's awareness, facilitates the conversation about QOL issues, and thus has been shown to be of value for doctor–patient communication (Detmar et al. 2002; Velikova et al. 2004; Velikova et al. 2010). Communication between doctor and patient is an essential aspect in the treatment of oncological patients. The majority of patients want support from their doctor. Thus, talking about QOL helps the doctor give the right kind of support. Patients receiving adequate information and who are content with the practitioner interaction, show a better QOL (Velikova et al. 2004).

In addition, evidence for a positive relationship between QOL data and duration of survival in cancer patients has been reported in different reviews (Gotay et al. 2008; Montazeri 2009; Quinten et al. 2009; Quinten et al. 2011). Thus, clinicians may benefit from the possible predictive value of QOL assessments in the treatment of cancer patients, as they may be used as early warning systems. Although patient and clinician ratings of clinical symptoms have been shown to differ, both are described as valuable in the estimation of overall survival (Quinten et al. 2011). Future research should examine whether and to what extent improvements in QOL have the potential to increase survival.

In palliative situations health care providers have the opportunity to effectively improve the QOL of their patients, especially in early stages of palliative care. Early support through specialized palliative interventions has been shown to lead to a greater improvement in QOL compared to usual care in patients newly diagnosed with non-small lung-cancer. Patients in the intervention group reported less depression and additionally showed a longer median survival (Temel et al. 2010).

A further issue of discussion is the facilitation of using QOL information for clinical doctors. Bezjak et al. (2001) recommend increasing the knowledge of oncologists on QOL literature by presenting findings in a comprehensible manner and emphasizing their clinical relevance. Furthermore doctors should address QOL issues and explore the patients' perceptions of QOL. Finally, the application and interpretation of QOL questionnaires should be facilitated, e.g., by using modern technology displaying clear and simple graphics with current and previous as well as normative QOL data.

4.3 Significance for People Affected by Cancer

In an European population-based survey ($n = 9344$) random households were asked what they would prioritize in the face of a serious illness like cancer: improving their QOL, prolonging survival or both. Across different countries, 57–81 % chose improving QOL, 2–6 % preferred extending life, and 15–40 % described both as being equally important (Higginson et al. 2013). Thus QOL issues seem to be of great value to the population.

Patients need to be informed about their disease, possible treatments, and the outcome of medical care. Information on the impact of a disease or treatment on their QOL is essential to patients especially while participating in decision making about the cancer care they undergo (Bottomley et al. 2005; Cella et al. 2002; de

Haes and Stiggelbout 1996). Both the psychosocial impairments (see "Psychosocial Impact of Cancer") and the worry and fear of recurrence or progression of the disease (see "Fear of progression") have a negative impact on QOL.

But also moving beyond active treatment, QOL remains an important topic for cancer survivors. Although cancer survivors have generally not been described as more vulnerable to the effects of day-to-day hassles, Costanzo et al. (2012) proposed a higher sensitivity to interpersonal tensions.

Cancer survivors may also be preoccupied with fears of recurrence, existential and spiritual problems, and experience difficulties in making new decisions considering their future life (Hewitt et al. 2005). Further challenges may be the adjustment to long-term and late effects like infertility and fatigue or changes in their social network, for example the loss of friendship due to the lack of support during treatment (Cella 1988). Each of these issues can have a major influence on QOL in the individual.

In a study with cervical cancer survivors ($n = 173$) 5, 10, and 15 years after diagnosis Le Borgne et al. (2013) showed a similarly good global QOL in cancer survivors compared to healthy controls. However, survivors 15 years after diagnosis reported more psychological burdens and—in case of prior radiotherapy—also more physical sequelae like sexual dysfunctions. Low income and comorbidities were further factors impairing QOL. Knowing different risk factors helps patients and health care professionals arrange appropriate interventions.

On the other hand it has been reported that cancer survivors often benefit from the cancer experience. A new appreciation of life, deeper spirituality, personal improvement, improved relationships, help orientation, and increased attention to their own health have been described as advantages of cancer survivorship in literature (Documet et al. 2012). An exploratory study with 39 breast cancer survivors 4.5–5 years after diagnosis showed that 2/3 described their lives as good or even better than before the diagnosis (Salander et al. 2011). Thus, cancer survival also seems to bring many opportunities to improve QOL (Hewitt et al. 2005). The development of a healthy lifestyle can give survivors a sense of control and more self-awareness as well as setting new priorities can help increase life satisfaction.

5   Challenges in Quality of Life-Measurements

A review of 794 randomized trials showed that in 25.4 % (200/794) HRQOL was a primary outcome (Brundage et al. 2011). Fourteen percent of the trials published their findings on QOL in a further publication. In general, the question remains, which and how many papers on QOL where actually accepted for publication (publication bias).

Planning and conducting clinical trials is associated with strict ethical requirements. How is the QOL of seriously ill people? Are patients with extremely impaired QOL even able to provide a realistic assessment of their situation? How do researchers deal with missing data? Missing data lead to less power, i.e., the fewer study participants, the lower the probability to detect differences.

Another possibility of bias in longitudinal assessments is the so-called response shift effect. In the context of QOL measurement and cancer patients, response shift implies changes in patients' internal standards, values, and understanding or perception of QOL while adapting to their disease and its treatment (Dabakuyo et al. 2013). Part of the psychological adaption in the process of disease for example may be a change in the patient's concept of 'worst pain imaginable'. Furthermore patients may set new priorities and develop a new concept of QOL (Luckett and King 2010). Thus, the correct interpretation of results in QOL measurement may require the assessment and adjustment for response shift effects.

More specific measurements assessing particular symptoms may be more responsive to change than a global measure of QOL. Further disadvantages of a global measure are its greater vulnerability to response shift effects and its inability to show changes in single dimensions of QOL. Nevertheless if the relative burden of one disease is to be compared with others, the assessment of overall QOL may be more appropriate and also more convenient (Luckett and King 2010).

Furthermore other sources of error in studies cannot be excluded: social desirability is a phenomenon which occurs repeatedly. There is a possibility that patients answer in ways not to offend their doctor. On the other hand patients may perceive QOL assessments as time-consuming and sometimes as an additional burden.

In literature one repeatedly encounters studies in which the QOL of cancer patients after treatment is compared with the QOL of healthy subjects due to missing control groups. It appears questionable if such comparisons are appropriate.

6 Quality of Life of Health Care Providers

The impact cancer has especially on the family of patients is described in "Psychosocial Burden of Family Caregivers to Adults with Cancer". But what would oncology be without the professional health care providers?

"Cancer is often seen as precipitating an existential crisis; a crisis of spirit and an opportunity for meaning. This is true not only for the patient with cancer and his or her family and loved ones, but also, interestingly enough, for oncologists and cancer care providers" (Breitbart 2006).

We have performed extensive literature searches on QOL. Alone the keyword search in PubMed "QOL and cancer" reveals over 43,700 entries. Health care providers appear only in the context of QOL-research, when it comes to observer-rated assessments of QOL of patients.

In a very impressive paper Laurie Lyckholm (2001) reports on handling stress, burnout, and grief in the practice of oncology. Causes of stress are seen in insufficient personal or vacation time, a sense of failure, unrealistic expectations, anger, frustration, as well as feelings of inadequacy or self preservations, reimbursement, and other issues related to managed care and third party payers, and last but not least grieving. Burnout can manifest itself in substance abuse, marital conflict, overeating and substantial weight gain, higher frequency of mistakes in clinical care, inappropriate emotional outbursts, interaction problems, depression and anxiety disorders, and even suicide. Lack of or inadequate training of communication and management skills are also considered causes of burnout (Ramirez et al. 1996). In a survey of 7,288 physicians in the United States, 45.8 % reported at least one of the following symptoms of burnout: loss of enthusiasm for work, feelings of cynicism (depersonalisation), and low sense of personal accomplishment (Shanafelt et al. 2012).

Thus, few but meaningful results on QOL of healthcare providers make further research in this area necessary, in order to provide effective interventions and strategies for these individuals. Ultimately, this would in turn be advantageous for the patients.

7 Summary

Cancer itself has a negative impact on the QOL of patients. However, individual conditions, values, and resources play an important role. Generally, and in various definitions HRQOL is considered as a multifactorial concept. In the assessment of QOL, observer-rated assessments were increasingly replaced by self-reports of patients. Meanwhile, validated assessment tools for different research questions and treatment settings exist in different languages. Many improvements have been made in QOL-research. However, there are still many trials with study designs of low quality (not randomized or prospective, etc.) and were QOL is missing as an outcome measure. Furthermore the variety of research results is often inconsistent, making it difficult to draw clear conclusions.

Nevertheless information on possible changes in QOL is not only relevant for researchers, as described above, but also has implications for clinicians and for people affected by cancer. Ideally, it forms a basis for shared decision making.

Last but not least more attention must be paid to the QOL of health care providers, which in turn would be beneficial to the patients and their families.

...and that's
  good enough reason to live... (The Wood Brothers 2006)

References

Archer VR, Billingham LJ, Cullen MH (1999) Palliative chemotherapy: no longer a contradiction in terms. Oncologist 4(6):470–477
Bertani E, Chiappa A, Biffi R et al (2011) Assessing appropriateness for elective colorectal cancer surgery: clinical, oncological, and quality-of-life short-term outcomes employing different treatment approaches. Int J Colorectal Dis 26(10):1317–1327
Bezjak A, Ng P, Skeel R et al (2001) Oncologists' use of quality of life information: results of a survey of eastern cooperative oncology group physicians. Qual Life Res 10(1):1–14

Bottomley A, Flechtner H, Efficace F et al (2005) Health related quality of life outcomes in cancer clinical trials. Eur J Cancer 41(12):1697–1709

Breitbart W (2006) Communication as a bridge to hope and healing in cancer care. In: Stiefel F (ed) Recent results in cancer research: communication in cancer care. Springer Berlin Heidelberg

Brundage M, Bass B, Davidson J et al (2011) Patterns of reporting health-related quality of life outcomes in randomized clinical trials: implications for clinicians and quality of life researchers. Qual Life Res 20(5):653–664

Calmann KC (1984) Quality of life in cancer patients—an hypothesis. J Med Ethics 10(3):124–127

Cella DF (1988) Quality of life during and after cancer treatment. Compr Ther 14(5):69–75

Cella DF, Tulsky DS, Gray G et al (1993) The functional assessment of cancer therapy scale: development and validation of the general measure. J Clin Oncol 11(3):570–579

Cella D, Hahn E, Dineen K (2002) Meaningful change in cancer-specific quality of life scores: Differences between improvement and worsening. Qual Life Res 11(3):207–221

Cella D, Gershon R, Lai J-S et al (2007) The future of outcomes measurement: item banking, tailored short-forms, and computerized adaptive assessment. Qual Life Res 16(1):133–141

Cocks K, King MT, Velikova G et al (2008) Quality, interpretation and presentation of European Organisation for Research and Treatment of Cancer quality of life questionnaire core 30 data in randomised controlled trials. Eur J Cancer 44(13):1793–1798

Cocks K, King MT, Velikova G et al (2011) Evidence-based guidelines for determination of sample size and interpretation of the European organisation for the research and treatment of cancer quality of life questionnaire core 30. J Clin Oncol 29(1):89–96

Cocks K, King MT, Velikova G et al (2012) Evidence-based guidelines for interpreting change scores for the European Organisation for the Research and Treatment of Cancer Quality of Life Questionnaire Core 30. Eur J Cancer 48(11):1713–1721

Costanzo ES, Stawski RS, Ryff CD et al (2012) Cancer survivors' responses to daily stressors: implications for quality of life. Health Psychol 31(3):360–370

Dabakuyo TS, Guillemin F, Conroy T et al (2013) Response shift effects on measuring post-operative quality of life among breast cancer patients: a multicenter cohort study. Qual Life Res 22(1):1–11

de Haes JCJM, Stiggelbout AM (1996) Assessment of values, utilities and preferences in cancer patients. Cancer Treat Rev 22A(0):13–26

de Ruiter MB, Reneman L, Boogerd W et al (2011) Cerebral hyporesponsiveness and cognitive impairment 10 years after chemotherapy for breast cancer. Hum Brain Mapp 32(8):1206–1219

Detmar S, Muller M, Schornagel J et al (2002) Health-related quality-of-life assessments and patient-physician communication: a randomized controlled trial. JAMA 288(23):3027–3034

Documet P, Trauth J, Key M et al (2012) Breast cancer survivors' perception of survivorship. Oncol Nurs Forum 39(3):309–315

Efficace F, Bottomley A, Osoba D et al (2003) Beyond the Development of Health-Related Quality-of-Life (HRQOL) Measures: A checklist for evaluating HRQOL outcomes in cancer clinical trials—does HRQOL evaluation in prostate cancer research inform clinical decision making? J Clin Oncol 21(18):3502–3511

Fallowfield L (2009) What is quality of life? In: http://www.medicine.ox.ac.uk/bandolier/painres/download/whatis/WhatisQOL.pdf

Fayers P, Bottomley A (2002) Quality of life research within the EORTC—the EORTC QLQ-C30. Euro J Cancer 38(Suppl 4 (0)):125–133

Fernández-Ortega P, Caloto MT, Chirveches E et al (2012) Chemotherapy-induced nausea and vomiting in clinical practice: impact on patients' quality of life. Support Care Cancer 20(12):3141–3148

Gotay CC, Kawamoto CT, Bottomley A et al (2008) The prognostic significance of patient-reported outcomes in cancer clinical trials. J Clin Oncol 26(8):1355–1363

Grumann M, Noack EM, Hoffmann I et al (2001) Comparison of quality of life in patients undergoing abdominoperineal extirpation or anterior resection for rectal cancer. Ann Surg 233(2):149–156

Haloua MH, Krekel N, Winters HAH et al (2013) A systematic review of oncoplastic breast-conserving surgery: current weaknesses and future prospects. Ann Surg 257(4):609–6020

Herschbach P (2002) Das "Zufriedenheitsparadox" in der Lebensqualitätsforschung. Psychother Psych Med 52(03/04):141–150

Hewitt M, Greenfield S, Stovall E (2005) From cancer patient to cancer survivor: lost in transition. The National Academies Press, Washington, DC

Higginson IJ, Gomes B, Calanzani N et al. (2013) Priorities for treatment, care and information if faced with serious illness: a comparative population-based survey in seven European countries. Palliat Med. doi:10.1177/0269216313488989

Jereczek-Fossa BA, Marsiglia HR, Orecchia R (2002) Radiotherapy-related fatigue. Crit Rev Oncol/Hematol 41(3):317–325

Kanellopoulos A, Hamre HM, Dahl AA et al (2013) Factors associated with poor quality of life in survivors of childhood acute lymphoblastic leukemia and lymphoma. Pediatr Blood Cancer 60(5):849–855

Karnofsky DA, Burchenal JH (1949) The clinical evaluation of chemotherapeutic agents in cancer. In: MacLeod CM (ed) Evaluation of chemotherapeutic agents. Columbia University Press, New York pp 196

King MT (1996) The interpretation of scores from the EORTC quality of life questionnaire QLQ-C30. Qual Life Res 5(6):555–567

King MT (2001) Cohen confirmed? Empirical effect sizes for the QLQ-C30. Qual Life Res 10(3):278

King PM, Blazeby JM, Ewings P et al (2006) Randomized clinical trial comparing laparoscopic and open surgery for colorectal cancer within an enhanced recovery programme. Br J Surg 93(3):300–308

Langius JAE, van Dijk AM, Doornaert P et al (2013) More than 10% weight loss in head and neck cancer patients during radiotherapy is independently associated with deterioration in quality of life. Nutr Cancer 65(1):76–83

Le Borgne G, Mercier M, Woronoff A-S et al (2013) Quality of life in long-term cervical cancer survivors: a population-based study. Gynecol Oncol 129(1):222–228

Leplège A, Hunt S (1997) The problem of quality of life in medicine. JAMA 278(1):47–50

Luckett T, King MT (2010) Choosing patient-reported outcome measures for cancer clinical research—Practical principles and an algorithm to assist non-specialist researchers. Eur J Cancer 46(18):3149–3157

Luckett T, King MT, Butow PN et al (2011) Choosing between the EORTC QLQ-C30 and FACT-G for measuring health-related quality of life in cancer clinical research: issues, evidence and recommendations. Ann Oncol 22(10):2179–2190

Lyckholm L (2001) Dealing with stress, burnout, and grief in the practice of oncology. Lancet Oncol 2(12):750–755

Mohamedali H, Breunis H, Timilshina N et al (2012) Older age is associated with similar quality of life and physical function compared to younger age during intensive chemotherapy for acute myeloid leukemia. Leuk Res 36(10):1241–1248

Montazeri A (2009) Quality of life data as prognostic indicators of survival in cancer patients: an overview of the literature from 1982 to 2008. Health and Qual Life Outcomes 7(1):102

Mrak K, Jagoditsch M, Eberl T et al (2011) Long-term quality of life in pouch patients compared with stoma patients following rectal cancer surgery. Colorectal Dis 13(12):403–410

Norman GR, Sloan JA, Wyrwich KW (2003) Interpretation of changes in health-related quality of life: the remarkable universality of half a standard deviation. Med Care 41(5):582–592

Osoba D (1994) Lessons learned from measuring health-related quality of life in oncology. J Clin Oncol 12(3):608–616

Osoba D (2011) Health-related quality of life and cancer clinical trials. Ther Adv Med Oncol 3(2):57–71

Osoba D, Rodrigues G, Myles J et al (1998) Interpreting the significance of changes in health-related quality-of-life scores. J Clin Oncol 16(1):139–144

Osoba D, Bezjak A, Brundage M et al (2005) Analysis and interpretation of health-related quality-of-life data from clinical trials: basic approach of The National Cancer Institute of Canada Clinical Trials Group. Eur J Cancer 41(2):280–287

Pachler J, Wille-Jorgensen P (2012) Quality of life after rectal resection for cancer, with or without permanent colostomy. Cochrane Database of Syst Rev 12:CD004323

Quinten C, Coens C, Mauer M et al (2009) Baseline quality of life as a prognostic indicator of survival: a meta-analysis of individual patient data from EORTC clinical trials. Lancet Oncol 10(9):865–871

Quinten C, Maringwa J, Gotay CC et al (2011) Patient self-reports of symptoms and clinician ratings as predictors of overall cancer survival. J Natl Cancer Inst 103(24):1851–1858

Ramirez AJ, Graham J, Richards MA et al (1996) Mental health of hospital consultants: the effects of stress and satisfaction at work. Lancet 347:724–728

Salander P, Lilliehorn S, Hamberg K et al (2011) The impact of breast cancer on living an everyday life 4.5–5 years post-diagnosis—a qualitative prospective study of 39 women. Acta Oncol 50(3):399–407

Schumacher M, Olschewski M, Schulgen G (1991) Assessment of quality of life in clinical trials. Stat Med 10(12):1915–1930

Scott-Brown M, Miah A, Harrington K et al (2010) Evidence-based review: quality of life following head and neck intensity-modulated radiotherapy. Radiother Oncol 97(2):249–257

Shanafelt TD, Boone S, Tan L et al (2012) Burnout and satisfaction with work-life balance among us physicians relative to the general us population. Arch Intern Med 172(18): 1377–1385

Spitzer WO, Dobson AJ, Hall J et al (1981) Measuring the quality of life of cancer patients: a concise QL-index for use by physicians. J Chronic Dis 34(12):585–597

Sprangers MAG, Cull A, Groenvold M et al (1998) The European organization for research and treatment of cancer approach to developing questionnaire modules: an update and overview. Qual Life Res 7(4):291–300

Temel JS, Greer JA, Muzikansky A et al (2010) Early palliative care for patients with metastatic non-small-lung-cancer. N Engl J Med 363:733–742

The Wood Brothers (2006) Chocolate on my tongue. In: Ways not to loose; http://www. songmeanings.com/songs/view/3530822107858616716

Veiga DF, Veiga-Filho J, Ribeiro LM et al (2010) Quality-of-life and self-esteem outcomes after oncoplastic breast-conserving surgery 125(3):811–817

Velikova G, Booth L, Smith AB et al (2004) Measuring quality of life in routine oncology practice improves communication and patient well-being: a randomized controlled trial. J Clin Oncol 22(4):714–724

Velikova G, Keding A, Harley C et al (2010) Patients report improvements in continuity of care when quality of life assessments are used routinely in oncology practice: secondary outcomes of a randomised controlled trial. Eur J Cancer 46(13):2381–2388

Weis J, Arraras JI, Conroy T et al (2013) Development of an EORTC quality of life phase III module measuring cancer-related fatigue (EORTC QLQ-FA13). Psycho-Oncology 22(5): 1002–1007

WHO (1946). In: Preamble to the Constitution of the World Health Organization as adopted by the International Health Conference, New York, 19–22 June, 1946; signed on 22 July 1946 by the representatives of 61 States (Official Records of the World Health Organization, no 2, p 100) and entered into force on 7 April 1948

WHO (1993) Study protocol for the World Health Organization project to develop a quality of life assessment instrument (WHOQOL). Qual Life Res 2(2):153–159

Printed by Books on Demand, Germany